.75

12 STEPS TO RAW FOODS

Additional praise for *12 Steps to Raw Foods*

"Starting from her own personal observations and experience, followed by her usual thorough research, Victoria Boutenko presents a wealth of information that challenges conventional thinking about the ideal human diet. I strongly recommend this highly readable book."
—Vance M. Logan, MD

"This book is a bible for the raw vegan."
—Ralph Anderson, quantum nutritional biochemist

"The thoroughness of Victoria Boutenko's research and the clarity of presentation is refreshing. From practical implementation of the diet and the wide range of healthy habits necessary for optimal health to addressing the deep-seated emotional and spiritual issues that can sabotage even the best thought-out raw program, she has covered it all. I will recommend this book to my patients, students, family, and friends."
—Ritamarie Loscalzo, DC, MS, CCN, DACBN

"Because of Victoria's 12-Step program, my family and I experience more out of life than we ever dreamed possible, with even more life force. Raw is the best way to be."
—Linda Bruno, medical herbalist, colonic hygienist, iridologist

Other books by Victoria Boutenko
Green for Life
Raw Family: A True Story of Awakening

12 Steps to
RAW
FOODS

How to End Your Dependency on Cooked Food

Victoria Boutenko, MA
Foreword by Gabriel Cousens, MD, MD(H)

North Atlantic Books
Berkeley, California

Published by
North Atlantic Books   Cover photo by Monika Adamczyk
P.O. Box 12327   Cover design by Claudia Smelser
Berkeley, California 94712   Book design by Brad Greene

Printed in the United States of America

12 Steps to Raw Foods: How to End Your Dependency on Cooked Food is sponsored by the Society for the Study of Native Arts and Sciences, a nonprofit educational corporation whose goals are to develop an educational and cross-cultural perspective linking various scientific, social, and artistic fields; to nurture a holistic view of arts, sciences, humanities, and healing; and to publish and distribute literature on the relationship of mind, body, and nature.

North Atlantic Books' publications are available through most bookstores. For further information, call 800-733-3000 or visit our website at www.northatlanticbooks.com.

Library of Congress Cataloging-in-Publication Data

Boutenko, Victoria.
    12 steps to raw foods : how to end your dependency on cooked food / by Victoria Boutenko. — Rev. and expanded ed.
        p. cm.
    Summary: "A revised and expanded version of the original, this book illuminates the average person's multi-level attachment to cooked foods, explains how one can successfully transition to a raw food diet, and—relying on new scientific evidence—explains the health benefits of eating raw, living foods"— Provided by publisher.
    Includes bibliographical references and index.
    ISBN-13: 978-1-55643-651-2
    ISBN-10: 1-55643-651-3
    1. Raw food diet. 2. Raw foods. I. Title.
TX353.B665 2007
613.2'6—dc22
                                                            2006100493
                                                            CIP

3 4 5 6 7 8 9 VERSA 14 13 12 11 10 09 08

To my mother, Valentina Boulgakova,
and my father, Valeri Gladkikh,
whom I love and miss deeply, and who continue
to inspire me even from the heavens.

*

Acknowledgments

I am grateful to my family for their ongoing love, patience, and support that I especially needed while writing this book.

My sincere thanks go to my angel helper, Christopher Sabatini, who took over my entire office work for several months, providing me with optimal conditions for a creative effort.

I am especially thankful to my friend, biochemist Ed Kellogg, PhD, for reading through the chapters containing scientific information.

I feel truly blessed with my friends who volunteered to spend many hours, sometimes at night, editing my manuscript: Victoria Bidwell, Laura Hamilton, Christopher Sabatini, Robert V. Grater, Verawnika Clay, and Caryne Palmer.

Finally, I would like to express my gratitude to Phyllis Linn, Lonny and Carmen Doi, Graham W. Boyes, and Pamela Joy for providing their generous financial support of my research during the months that I dedicated to writing this book and did not lecture.

Thank you, dear friends. May you always be blessed with health, joy, love, and prosperity!

Contents

Foreword to the Second Edition of
12 Steps to Raw Foods

The first edition of this book (published in 2000) was excellent. The second edition is *masterfully outstanding*. In the last six years, Victoria Boutenko has established a fresh outlook on nutrition and revealed herself as a live-food woman of wisdom. She offers tremendous insights on the benefits of raw foods. Her studies of the importance of greens in the human diet are particularly interesting and constitute a breakthrough for the live-food movement. Her work using blended greens is valuable both as a transition diet for people with a very poor digestive system, and as general nutritional support for just about anyone consuming the greens at least once a day. Victoria highlights the importance of greens by explaining how she attained a high level of health by adding a sufficient amount of greens to her live-food diet.

Victoria successfully conveys the significance of live foods. The depth of her book is marked not only by copious new research on the benefits of raw foods, but by a clarity that shines through these pages—the clarity of her own soul. Victoria's wisdom and understanding of the live-foods lifestyle is communicated with enthusiasm and pointedness.

Scientifically, she shares many interesting facts that have only become available in recent years—for example, her excellent research on how humans went from a raw, primarily vegan diet (similar to that of the chimpanzee) to a meat-eating diet.

Victoria's review of the research on advanced glycoxidation end products (AGEs) is particularly relevant because AGEs play a major part in the degeneration process when there is an excess amount of sugar in the system. A high level of AGEs in the diet can lead to neurodegeneration, cardiovascular problems, and kidney failure. As we see with diabetes, the AGEs are literally a form of accelerated aging.

It is really gratifying to see the level of documentation and research of scientific journals that Victoria provides throughout her book. Victoria mentions research about acrylamide—a carcinogenic substance associated with cooked starches. This is now a global problem, since acrylamide seems to be considered a carcinogen for humans. Cooked and processed meats and fish create heterocyclic amines, along with other mutagens and carcinogens. So obviously we avoid all of these toxins when we eat live foods.

Victoria also brings to light lots of scientific studies that illustrate the presence of multiple beneficial elements in living foods, such as phytonutrients and antioxidants, as well as many others. For example, molecules of resveratrol can activate human longevity genes, and falcarinol in raw carrots aids in preventing and healing cancer.

Overall, *12 Steps to Raw Foods* is a breakthrough work for the live-food movement. One important point Victoria Boutenko humbly and with great wisdom articulates in this book is the fact that some people are dependent on cooked foods, for the variety of reasons she talks about. Because of this addiction, it is difficult to transition gracefully to a full live-food diet. Victoria outlines a clear solution to this problem with her 12-Step program. People need a lot of support to move into live foods, and they also need a thoughtful and compassionate program to support them after the initial decision. This book, *12 Steps to Raw Foods*, helps significantly. Victoria fills her 12 Steps with really practical information and insight for the transition.

Before reading this book in 2000 and talking with Victoria about it, I did not fully understand the addictive power of cooked foods. I applaud Victoria for this breakthrough. I am happy that this book is on the market, and I recommend it to all who come to the Tree of Life Rejuvenation Center (a live-food center and oasis for awakening located in the mountains of southern Arizona where I am Director). This second edition is so much deeper that I am now also recommending it to my staff as mandatory reading so that they can be much more understanding, compassionate, and insightful about live foods.

Victoria's genuine humility and wisdom make this book even more powerful. By sharing the stories of her own transition and some of the difficulties in her family, the author gives us a very personal and heartfelt book. Victoria takes a good look at cultural attachment, social pressures, programming from birth, and addictive qualities of processed food, then gives people ways to deal with these problems so they can succeed in making changes. The stories of her family's struggles and the growth they have experienced in this process are truly a human inspiration, as well as a live-food one for the community.

While the most important contribution of this book is likely to be the clear insight that cooked food may be an addiction, Victoria also gives an in-depth overview of the importance of live foods for our health and well-being. She shares insights about live-food preparation, particularly her green smoothies. She focuses less on the recipes than on understanding how to play with the food in a way that encourages us to make our own creations, simply and in the manner that best meets our needs. Victoria's raw-food woman's wisdom gives the reader a sophisticated understanding of the ins and outs of transitioning to live foods. Like we try to do at the Tree of Life, she makes the point that raw food should be delicious, particularly in the beginning, because people need the psychological comfort of gourmet quality to make their transition. At the same time, she points out what most raw-food enthusiasts eventually learn: the more we are involved in the raw-food way of life, the less we need the gourmet level except perhaps at parties. Victoria gives people gems to which they can hang on to help them succeed in becoming raw-food people.

Another positive aspect of this book is its support for turning people into their own best expert. As the author points out, there is a lot of confusion in the nutrition field, live food or not, and Victoria's approach is to encourage people—once they are through the detoxification—to trust their own body cravings, because these cravings often tell us what we really need for our specific body health at the moment.

This book is a classic. I appreciate the opportunity to write the foreword to the second edition. I emphatically recommend *12 Steps to Raw Foods* to anyone who is involved in helping people move into a live-food lifestyle, to any teacher of live foods, and to any live-food friend who needs support. Victoria's book is one of the most supportive, nurturing, and wise offerings in the live-food movement that I have seen in years. I am very grateful for the breakthrough and the wisdom that she shares. Blessings to your health, well-being, and spiritual joy.

—Gabriel Cousens, MD, MD(H)
Diplomat, American Board of Holistic Medicine
Diplomat in Ayurveda
Director of the Tree of Life Rejuvenation Center
Author of *Spiritual Nutrition, Conscious Eating,* and *Rainbow Green Live Food Cuisine*

Author's Note

I believe that we are all designed to be healthy, that our beautiful bodies are perfect, and that sickness is not normal. Yet how many people can you name who are absolutely healthy? I understand that our health and liveliness largely depend on nutrition. Most of us have at least some idea about which foods can make us healthy and energized. I associate being healthy with feeling an enjoyable lightness in my body, having a pleasant mood, and thinking clearly, but most importantly, having the energy to manifest my *dreams*. I remember how my former sickness eliminated much of the joy from my life; it drained my energy and kept me from doing the activities that would have made me most happy and fulfilled.

In our society, it is common to entertain the hopeless belief that a lot of illnesses are incurable. I contend that for many people this belief is based in a dependence on unhealthy foods and a feeling of being unable to change our eating habits. Unfortunately, doctors are powerless to compensate for this lack of nutrition, even though they do all they know to help.

Every day I observe people around me who are desperate to improve their nutrition but are still unable to change their habits. They find themselves—time and again—eating what they so resolutely had planned to avoid. Through much experimenting and research, I have come to the conclusion that becoming free from this dependency is possible, and that managing one's diet can drastically improve one's health.

Over the past twelve years, I have taught thousands of classes and weekend workshops worldwide. I receive "Thank You" letters from the thousands of people who have used my coping techniques to successfully eat healthier. In this revised and expanded edition of *12 Steps to Raw Foods,* I have updated my research with the latest scientific data; I have added more of my personal experiences; I have addressed historical issues such as how the human dependency on cooked food formed; and I have included my most successful coping techniques, along with my most delicious recipes.

Enjoy this reading—I look forward to running into you at a juice bar!

In Good Health,

—Victoria

Part 1

WHY RAW FOOD?

Chapter 1

WHERE MY SEARCH BEGAN

"Ask, and it shall be given you; seek, and ye shall find; knock, and it shall be opened unto you."

—Matthew 7:7

We joke in my family that we were fortunate to get sick all together, but back then, in 1993, our health problems were no joke. All four of us (my husband, our two children, and me) were deathly sick. I was only thirty-eight, and I was already diagnosed with the same disease that took my father, arrhythmia, which is an irregular heartbeat. My legs were constantly swollen from edema; I weighed 280 pounds; and I was continuing to gain more weight. My left arm frequently became numb at night, and I was afraid that I would die and my children would become orphans. I remember always feeling tired and depressed. At last, my doctor told me that there was nothing else she could do for my health. She said, "I think you just have to pray now."

My husband, Igor, had been frequently ill since his early childhood. By the tender age of seventeen, he had already survived nine surgeries. Having progressive hyperthyroidism and chronic rheumatoid arthritis, by age thirty-eight he was a total health wreck. I had to lace his shoes on rainy days because his arthritic spine would not bend. Igor's heart rate was 140+ most of the time, his eyes were tearing on sunny days, and his hands were shaky. Igor constantly felt fatigued and in pain. His doctor told him to prepare to spend the rest of his life in a wheelchair.

Our daughter Valya was born with asthma and allergies. She was a pale, pasty girl, leading a sedentary lifestyle because she would start coughing and choking as soon as she ran or jumped. In 1993, at the age of eight, Valya woke up almost every night with a cough that wouldn't stop until Igor gave her a drainage massage.

Finally, our son Sergei, who was nine, was diagnosed with diabetes. We were already spending two to four thousand dollars a month on our medical bills, insurance, doctors' appointments and prescriptions, when in September of 1993 the doctors told us that Sergei needed to go on insulin.

Igor and I were shocked. My diabetic grandmother had recently passed away from an overdose of insulin. I couldn't imagine putting Sergei on this powerful drug. I remember sitting in the kitchen crying that whole night through, asking, "God, why do you punish my family? What did we do wrong? How much more can we handle? Why is our health getting worse and worse, in spite of all our efforts?" I kept saying, "I cannot put him on insulin. I just can't."

In the morning I went to the medical library and checked out several books on diabetes. All of these books explained that insulin shots would eventually weaken Sergei's eyesight and could cause kidney failure. Now my fear of insulin grew even stronger. I didn't know what to do, so I decided to procrastinate. I was hoping to be able to postpone Sergei's insulin treatments for two weeks or more while I looked for a solution. My grandmother used to repeat, "Seek and you shall find." With these words in my heart, I began actively searching for a solution.

I kept my eyes and ears open all the time. I started asking everyone I met about alternative treatments for diabetes. After scaring numerous people, I figured out that it made sense to ask only those people who looked healthy. I became pretty good at spotting healthy-looking individuals on the street and developed my own approach. First I told the fit-looking stranger, "Oh, you look radiantly healthy." Normally they would smile and say, "Thank you!" Then I asked them about diabetes. At first I got trapped by several sales reps; in one week, I had a thick stack of business cards from different companies that sold supplements or offered alternative treatments. I had no idea what I was looking for, but I kept searching.

In two months' time, a miracle happened! The universe placed before me a raw-fooder who lived in Colorado at that time. Elizabeth was standing in front of me in line at my bank, just two blocks from my home. When I looked at her, I understood firsthand what people mean when they say "glowing skin"! I told her that she looked radiantly healthy and asked her, "Do you think one can heal diabetes naturally?"

She shone at me with her smile. "Sure!"

"Why are you so sure?" I eagerly inquired.

"Because I cured my colon cancer, stage four, twenty years ago," Elizabeth readily offered.

"But it's not the same as having diabetes!" I protested.

"Oh yes, it's all the same," Elizabeth firmly corrected me.

"Can I please buy you lunch so we can talk?" I pleaded.

"Thank you, but I won't eat your food. I will gladly answer your questions," Elizabeth obliged me.

Elizabeth and I sat outside the bank, and she told me about raw food. At first, I was disappointed. I was looking for a more serious solution. I was willing to work hard and pay any amount of money for some miraculous herb or treatment. Raw food sounded absurd to me—too simplistic. I'd heard of raw foods before, but I was not so naïve to believe that kind of stuff. So I asked Elizabeth, "Do you really believe that humans can survive on just fruits, vegetables, nuts and seeds, raw?!"

Elizabeth responded with three indisputable arguments: (1) animals do not cook; (2) I have been eating only raw food for twenty years and healed my colon cancer; (3) you did not come into this world with a cooking stove attached to your belly.

These points were far from being scientific, but I couldn't think of anything to refute them. Besides, I was greatly impressed with Elizabeth's youthful look, and I desperately wanted everyone in my family to feel better. Elizabeth loaned me a book about raw food and gave me her phone number. I went home and started reading the book.

I would like to point out that in 1993 there were only a few books about raw food available and they were not sold in stores, only by the authors themselves. I quickly read the book that Elizabeth loaned me, and suddenly the promises of the raw-food diet seemed obvious. Next, I became scared. I thought, "Now I have to give up the last pleasure that I have left in life." At the same time, I was already eager to try raw food and see if it would work.

Igor noticed my anxiety. He asked me, "What is that you're reading?"

I said, "Honey, I think I've found what will help our son—the raw-food diet! But I don't think he can do it alone. Igor, can we please try it as a family for just a couple of weeks to see if it works, please?"

Igor became very angry. "I am a Russian man, and I cannot live on rabbit food. I work physically. I love my Russian borscht with pork! Plus, food unites family. Dinner is the only time our family gets together. Now you want us to meet around carrot sticks?! Think a little. One has to study fourteen years to become a doctor! Do you think you know more than doctors do? Think of all the billions of dollars the government spends on medical research. Are you saying that they don't know anything and you do? If becoming healthy were so easy, doctors would have done it long ago. You know how much I love you. But if you are going to go on that crazy diet, you must realize that a divorce will be inevitable."

I was disappointed, but I decided to get back to the subject of raw food at a more appropriate time.

One morning my husband woke up feeling worse than ever before. He had a big swelling on his neck; he was in pain and couldn't talk. I took him to the hospital. After looking at Igor's new blood test, the doctor told him, "You need to have surgery. Your thyroid is no good anymore and needs to come out."

Igor protested, "I've already had nine surgeries. None of them helped me, and I have decided not to ever have another surgery in my life."

"This surgery is unavoidable," the doctor declared.

"What if I refuse?" Igor replied defiantly.

"Then you will die," the doctor calmly explained.

Igor inquired, "How soon?"

The doctor predicted, "Probably in less than two months."

"I will go on raw food instead!" Igor proclaimed.

We left. Little did we know that this day, January 21st of 1994, would mark the turning point in our family health history. Later

7

that day my husband, our two youngest children, and I went on a diet of raw food as a family and have been eating only raw food ever since. However, while we were driving home from the hospital we were not aware of our destiny as yet and agreed to try a raw-food diet for two weeks to see if there would be any improvement in our health at all.

A couple of hours later, when Igor left for work, I went into the kitchen. I fully realized that this could be the only chance in a life-time to make such a drastic change. Therefore, I was decisive. I carefully examined the food that we had in the fridge and in the cupboards and discovered that we had almost zero raw food in our house. Everything had to go! I took a heavy-duty garbage bag and cleaned out all the beans, macaroni, cereal, rice, TV dinners, popsicles, whipped cream, breads, sauces, cheese, and cans of tuna. Next went the coffeemaker, toaster, and pasta maker. I turned off the pilot light and covered the stove with a large cutting board. Now our kitchen looked as if we were moving out. The only item left on the counter was our huge, expensive microwave oven. When we lived in Russia, we couldn't have one because Russian scientists performed research and found out that microwave ovens are very harmful. For this reason microwave ovens were prohibited in Russia. As a result, when we came to the United States, we bought a big one. Now I was staring at this microwave oven and realized that I didn't know what to do about it. I started thinking about delicious melted cheese sandwiches, Pop Tarts, and all the "miracles" I used to bake in it. Then, I thought about Sergei and his diabetes. Most of all in the world, I did not want him to go on insulin. So I got a hammer and cracked the microwave's glass door. Then I put it in the garage. I took all our brand-new pots and pans (that I'd just gotten for Christmas) out onto the sidewalk, and they disappeared minutes later. Then I rushed to the local supermarket.

I was not aware at that time of the existence of raw gourmet dishes. I didn't know what raw-fooders ate, having never met any besides Elizabeth, who ate simply. I had never heard of dehydrated flax crackers, nut milks, seed cheese, or raw cakes. I thought of raw food as mainly being salads. Furthermore, I came from Russia, where fresh fruits and vegetables were available only during the summer. We were used to eating potatoes, meat, macaroni, lots of dairy products, and occasionally fruit. We were not accustomed to eating salads, and my family didn't like vegetables. Therefore, I was confined to merely the fruit section of the produce department. Due to our tight budget, we usually bought only Washington apples, naval oranges, and bananas. I loaded my cart with these three items.

When my kids came home from school and Igor from work, they asked, "What's for dinner?" I told them to look in the fridge. My children couldn't believe their eyes. "Where are our TV dinners? Where did all the ice cream go?" They threw a fit.

Sergei said, "I would rather take insulin shots for the rest of my life than stay on such a crazy diet." They refused to eat and went to their rooms to watch videos.

Igor ate a couple of bananas and complained that this food made him hungrier. We had lots of time that day. I remember everyone walking from one room to another looking at the clock. This was my initial realization of how much of my time had been spent thinking about, planning, preparing to eat, eating, and cleaning up afterwards. We felt hungry, uncomfortable, weird, and lost. We tried watching TV, but the grilled chicken commercials were unbearable. We hardly made it to nine o'clock. Unable to fall asleep due to my own empty stomach, I heard footsteps in our kitchen and the sound of drawers opening and closing.

In the morning, we woke up unusually early and gathered in the kitchen. I noticed lots of peels from bananas and oranges on the counter. Valya shared with us that she hadn't coughed that night. I remember telling her, "That is just a coincidence; the diet couldn't work that fast." Sergei checked his blood sugar. It was still high, but *it was lower* than it had been for several weeks. Igor and I noticed a slight energy increase, and generally, we felt lighter and more positive. We were also very hungry.

I have never told anyone that shifting to a raw-food diet is easy. In fact, it was very hard for the four of us. Our bodies were demanding foods that we used to eat. From the very first day, and for a couple weeks, minute after minute, I daydreamed of eating bagels with cream cheese, hot soups, chocolate, or at the very least, various types of chips. At night in my sleep, I was searching for French fries under my pillow. I sneaked two dollars from our family budget and kept them in my pocket. I kept plotting that one day, I would have half an hour alone to run down to the corner restaurant and buy a slice of hot, cheesy pizza, eat it fast without being seen, run back, and continue the raw-food diet. Luckily, I never found that chance.

Meanwhile, positive changes rapidly appeared. Valya stopped coughing at night and never had an asthmatic attack again. Sergei's blood sugar steadily began to stabilize. Igor's swelling in his throat subsided to normal. His pulse went down, and the symptoms of hyperthyroidism became less apparent with each day. I noticed that my clothes were loose on my body, even when they were fresh out of the dryer. That had never happened before. I was excited! Every morning, I ran to the mirror and examined my face, counting the disappearing wrinkles. My face definitely looked better and younger with each day of the raw life.

After one month on raw food, Sergei asked me why he had to check his blood sugar every three hours when it was now consistently within the normal range. I told him to check it only once, in the morning. Igor's pulse was down to 90, where it had not been for years. Valya was able to run a quarter of a mile at school without coughing. I lost fifteen pounds. All of us noticed that we had a lot more energy. I myself had so much energy that I could not walk anymore—I was always running! I ran from the parking lot to the store and between the aisles and up and down the stairs in our house. We had to come up with some exercise that would channel the extra energy we now had.

I once read that running is a must for diabetics.[1] The author explained that while exercising, the muscles produce additional insulin. We decided to start running as a family. Eventually, Sergei's blood sugar stabilized due to his new diet and regular jogging. From the day that we began to eat raw food to the present, he has never again experienced any form of diabetic symptoms.

In order to encourage my children to keep jogging, I signed my family up for a race. Since we had never run before, I chose the shortest race I could possibly find. It was a "Tiny Trot" run, one kilometer long, in Denver's Washington Park. When we arrived at the race, we found ourselves surrounded by very small children, but Sergei and Valya didn't seem to notice. Red and puffy, all four of us managed to reach the finish line. We were greeted by a crowd of parents, and each one of us received a medal for "First Place in Your Age Group"—the first athletic awards in our lives. My children were so happy, they refused to take off the medals for a week;

they even slept with them on. They begged me to sign them up for more races, and I did. From that point on, we were racing almost every weekend.

On Memorial Day that year, four months after we went raw, we ran the Bolder Boulder Race, a ten-kilometer run with forty thousand other runners. As we were running among healthy-looking people, many of whom were experienced runners, it was hard for us to imagine that only four months ago, we considered ourselves hopelessly ill. Each one of us came to the finish line with a satisfactory time, and we were not tired. After finishing the race, we went hiking in the mountains. We now had no doubts that our health was connected to our diet, and I knew that I was not dying from any disease because how could I run ten kilometers if I were dying?

We appreciated that our health was quickly restored to normal and that we had become even healthier than ever before. To share the story of our amazing healing with as many people as possible, and to inspire others to try this dietary approach, we have published a book entitled *Raw Family* (see Bibliography at back of book).

Chapter 2

WHAT WAS MISSING IN OUR RAW FOOD PLAN?

"Mistakes are the portals of discovery."

—James Joyce

My family fell into many pitfalls while staying on a raw-food diet. After several years of being raw-foodists, each one of us began to feel like we had reached a plateau where our healing processes stopped and even began to go backwards. After approximately seven years on a completely raw diet, once in a while, more and more often, we started feeling discontent with our existing food program. I began to have a heavy feeling in my stomach after eating almost any kind of raw food, especially a salad with dressing. Because of that, I started to eat fewer greens and more fruits and nuts. I began to gain weight. My husband started to develop a lot of gray hair.

My family members felt confused about our diet and seemed often to have the question, "What should we eat?" There were odd times when we felt hungry but did not desire any foods that were "legal" for us to eat on a typical raw-food diet: vegetables, fruits, nuts, seeds, grains, sprouts, or dried fruit. Salads (with dressings) were delicious but made us tired and sleepy. We felt trapped. I remember Igor looking inside the fridge, saying over and over again, "I wish I wanted some of this stuff." Such periods did not last. We blamed it all on stress and overeating and were able to refresh our appetites by fasts, exercise, hikes, or by working more. In my family we strongly believe that raw food is the *only way to go*. Therefore, we encouraged each other to maintain our raw diet no matter what, always coming up with new tricks. Many of my friends told me about similar experiences, at which point they gave up being 100% raw and began to add cooked food back into their meals. In my family, we continued to stay on raw food due to our constant support of each other.

A burning question began to grow stronger in my heart with each day. The question was, "Is there anything missing in our diet?" The answer would come right away: "Nope. Nothing could be better than a raw-food diet. This diet saved our lives."

Yet, however tiny, the unwanted signs of less than perfect health kept surfacing in minor but noticeable symptoms, such as a wart on a hand or a gray hair on the scalp—symptoms that brought doubts and questions about the completeness of the raw-food diet in its present form. Finally, when my children complained about the increased sensitivity of their teeth, I reached a state where I couldn't think about anything other than this health puzzle. I drove everybody around me crazy with my constant discussion of what could possibly be missing.

Chapter 3

ODE TO A GREEN SMOOTHIE

"And God said, Behold, I have given you every herb . . . upon the face of all the earth, . . . to you it shall be for food."

—Genesis 1:29

In my eager quest, I started collecting data about every single food that existed for humans. As my grandmother used to say, "Seek and ye shall find." After many wrong guesses, I finally found the correct answer. It was August 2004, ten years since my family had become raw-fooders and three years after we reached the plateau period.

I found one particular food group that matched *all* nutritional human needs: *greens*. The truth is, in my family we were not eating enough greens. Moreover, we did not like them. We knew that greens were important, but we had never heard anywhere exactly how many greens we needed in our diet. We had only a vague recommendation to eat as much as possible. In order to find out how many greens we needed to eat, I decided to study the eating habits of chimpanzees, since they are one of the closest creatures to human beings. Chimps consume 40% greens: that corresponds to two bunches of greens per day from the supermarket displays for us humans.

In my research, I noticed that chimpanzees really *love* greens. I remember watching chimps at the zoo and seeing how excited they became when given fresh acacia branches, young tender palm tree leaves, or kale. I was so inspired looking at them that I went to the nearby bushes and tried to eat acacia leaves myself. But the truth was, the green leaves were not very palatable for me and that presented another problem: Eating greens always seemed like a duty for me. I would think to myself, "I have to have my greens." Some days I would "cheat" by juicing my greens. I would quickly drink a cup of green juice and consider myself good for a couple of days. Or I would make a delicious raw dressing and sink my greens into it. That was another way for me to enjoy greens. But I could never imagine sitting and eating kale or spinach, plain, handful after handful.

I looked at the nutritional content of dozens of different green vegetables, and I was pleased to see that greens are rich in almost all essential minerals and vitamins recommended by USDA, including protein. I became convinced that greens are the most important food for humans. If I could only find a way to enjoy them enough to consume the optimal quantity needed to become perfectly healthy!

I tried countless times to force myself to eat large amounts of greens in the form of salad or by themselves, only to discover that I was not physically able to do that. After about two cups of shredded greens, I would have either heartburn or nausea.

One day while studying a book on biology, I became intrigued by the amazingly hardy composition of plants. Apparently cellulose, the main constituent of plants, has one of the strongest molecular structures on the planet. Greens possess more valuable nutrients than any other food group, but all these nutrients are stored inside the cells of plants. These cells are made of tough material, as a means of survival for the plant. The sturdy stems and leaves of greens allow them to stand up against winds and rains.

Greens make up the main diet for many animals. **To release all the valuable nutrients from within the cells, the cell walls need to be ruptured.** To rupture these sturdy cells is not easy. This is why eating greens without masticating them thoroughly would not satisfy our nutritional needs. In simple words, we need to chew our greens to a creamy consistency in order to get the benefits.

In addition, in order to digest the released minerals and vitamins, hydrochloric acid in the stomach has to be very strong, with a pH between 1 and 2.

These two conditions are necessary for the assimilation of nutrients from greens. Obviously, when I tried to eat plain greens, I did not chew them well enough, and possibly I did not have a high enough level of hydrochloric acid in my stomach. As a result, I experienced unpleasant signs of indigestion and formed a general dislike for greens altogether.

After many decades of eating mostly heavily processed foods, many modern people have lost their ability to chew normally.[1] For some, the jaws have become so narrow that even after having their wisdom teeth extracted, many people still need to wear braces to reduce crowding of the teeth.[2] Also, jaw muscles can become too weak to thoroughly chew rough fiber. Several times I have heard recommendations from my dentist to be more gentle on my teeth and not to bite firm fruit, but rather to grate my carrots and apples. In addition to these compromising conditions, many people have lots of fillings, dentures, or missing teeth. All of these obstacles make chewing greens to the necessary consistency virtually impossible.

This is why I decided to try to "chew" my greens in the Vita-Mix blender.* First I blended a bunch of kale with water. I was thinking, "I'll just close my eyes, hold my nose, and drink it." But as soon as I opened the lid, I closed it again quickly because I felt queasy from the strong wheatgrass smell. That dark-green, almost black mixture was totally unconsumable. After some brainstorming, I added several bananas and blended it again. And that was when the magic began! I slowly, and with some trepidation, removed the lid and sniffed the air, and to my great surprise, this bright-green concoction smelled very pleasant. I cautiously tasted a sip and was exhilarated! It was better than tasty! Not too sweet, not too bitter, it was the most unusual taste I had ever tried, and I could describe it in one word: "freshness."

In four hours I had consumed all I blended, which was one bunch of kale, four bananas, and a quart of water. I felt wonderful and made more. Triumphantly, I realized that this evening was the first time in my life that I had consumed two good-sized bunches of greens in one day. Plus, I ate them without any oil or salt! And I enjoyed the whole experience. My stomach felt fine, and I was happy to have achieved my goal.

---

*I would like to explain that the Vita-Mix is not just a simple blender like the ones you can find at any department store. It is called a "high-speed blender," because its speed goes up to 240 mph! That means that its blades don't even have to be sharp; they could be dull metal sticks and still liquefy something as hard as a block of wood. In order to reach such performance, the Vita-Mix has a 2+ peak horsepower motor. Any simple blender will blend the tough cellulose of greens only so long as its blades are sharp. Unfortunately, when the blades become dull, they just move around pieces of banana and the blender very quickly overheats. Eleven years ago, after burning out several blenders, I finally bought myself a Vita-Mix at the country fair. It still works like new.

The solution to my greens dilemma was so unexpectedly simple. To consume greens in this way took so little time that I naturally continued experimenting with blended greens and fruits day after day.

I must admit here that the idea of blended greens was not new to me.

Eleven years ago when my family was studying at the Creative Health Institute (CHI) in Michigan, we learned about the extraordinary healing properties of energy soup: blended sprouts, avocado, and apple. This soup was invented by Dr. Ann Wigmore, the pioneer of the Living Foods lifestyle in the twentieth century.* Although we were told countless times how exceptionally beneficial energy soup is, most of the guests at the institute were not able to swallow more than a couple of spoonfuls of energy soup because it was not palatable.

I was very impressed with the testimonials that I heard from people about the benefits of energy soup. When I returned home, I desperately experimented with energy soup, trying to improve the taste because I wanted my family to benefit from consuming it. My final attempt to perfect energy soup was ended one day when I heard Valya yelling to Sergei in the back yard, "Run! Mom is making that green mush again!"

Despite all the evidence of the healing powers of energy soup, unfortunately I found that even people who desperately needed and wanted it could not make themselves consume it regularly.

I am amazed that eleven years after being introduced to energy

---

*Dr. Ann Wigmore, DD, ND (1909–1993)—humanitarian, educator, and writer. Dr. Ann Wigmore designed and promoted a *Living Foods Lifestyle*.

soup, when I had completely forgotten about it, I came back to the very same idea of blended greens from an entirely new direction. When I first started drinking green smoothies, I didn't mention it to anybody and did not expect anything significant to happen. Since I did not have any big health problems at the time, I was not pursuing any dramatic changes. I just didn't want to age so noticeably. However, after about a month of erratic green smoothie drinking, two moles and a wart I had since early childhood peeled off my body. I felt more energized than ever before and started sharing my experience with my family and friends. My nails became stronger, my vision sharpened, and I had a wonderful taste in my mouth, even upon waking in the morning (a pleasure I hadn't enjoyed since youth).

My dream had come true at last! I was consuming plenty of greens every day. I began to feel lighter, and my energy increased. My tastes started to change. I discovered that my body was so starved for greens that for several weeks I lived almost entirely on green smoothies. Plain fruits and vegetables became much more desirable to me, and my cravings for fatty foods declined dramatically. I stopped consuming any kind of salt altogether, even seaweed.

Once, my husband and I were walking in California along a grassy trail when I suddenly began to salivate from looking at the dark-green, crispy branches of malva weeds growing in abundance along our path. I kept catching myself wanting to grab and eat them. I shared my observations with Igor, and he listened attentively but didn't get excited. He had already noticed that I was eating differently lately. Instead of making myself a huge salad consisting of multiple chopped vegetables, a large avocado, sea salt, lots of onion, and olive oil, I now chopped a bunch of lettuce with a tomato, sprinkled it with lemon juice, and enjoyed it tremendously, rolling my eyes and humming with pleasure. I did not miss my former food and felt completely satisfied eating so simply. Now I knew that the human body can learn to crave greens!

Yet another change astounded me. I used to have cravings for unhealthy foods when I would get tired. For example, in the past, when we had been traveling and spent the night in an airplane, or after driving all night, I experienced severe cravings for heavy raw foods or even some authentic Russian cooked foods from childhood that I hadn't eaten for more than a decade. These cravings were very strong and annoying. Driven by these urges, I would prepare myself some kind of dense raw food, like seed cheese with crackers, or I'd stuff myself with nuts, sometimes late at night. I have heard from many other people that they experienced similar patterns. Also, during previous years, when I came home late from my office, often after ten p.m., I enjoyed changing my focus from work to lighter topics, either by reading a chapter from a book or by watching a nice video. I noticed that if I allowed myself to grab an apple or a handful of nuts, I would tend to continue grazing and couldn't ever achieve a feeling of satisfaction. Even if I used my will power and didn't touch any food at home, I continued to feel discontent and to think about food.

When I began to drink green smoothies, I noticed right away that those cravings disappeared. That was when my husband really noticed the difference in my behavior. In the evening after a hard work day, he would still crave something to eat while I was relaxed and content by just reading a book or talking. When Igor saw how happy I was in the evenings, along with the noticeable improvements in my health, he joined me in drinking green smoothies. He started to ask for a cup of "that green stuff" whenever I was making it.

Soon, both Igor and I were able to testify that we experienced rejuvenation. Our cravings for the heavy foods stopped. After only two months of drinking smoothies, Igor's mustache and beard started growing in blacker, making him look like he did when we first met.

Igor was so enthusiastic about his youthful look that he became the green-smoothie champion of my family. He woke up early and made two or three gallons of smoothie every day: one for me, one for him, and one for Sergei and Valya to share. Both children enjoyed including this tasty green drink in their daily menu even though they were already experiencing great health. They noticed still more benefits, like the ability to sleep less, more complete eliminations, stronger nails, and most of all, improvement in their teeth and gums.

Now I couldn't imagine my life without my green smoothies, as they had become a staple of my diet. In addition to smoothies, I ate flax crackers, salads, fruit, and occasionally seeds or nuts. In order to always have the opportunity to make fresh green smoothies for myself, I purchased an additional Vita-Mix blender for my office. Whenever friends or customers came in, they saw a big green cup next to my computer; and I treated them to a sample of my new discovery. To my great satisfaction, everybody loved it, despite their different dietary habits. Even the UPS guy liked it.

Inspired by the warm reception, I wrote an article about my new experience and emailed it to everyone in my Internet address book. Almost instantly, I began receiving strong, positive feedback and many detailed testimonials from my friends, students, and customers. The number of people drinking green smoothies turned into a "green wave," growing rapidly every day. Based on research that I have done, I consider green smoothies to be the greatest source of nourishment for humans. Below I list ten of the many benefits of green smoothies.

Ten Benefits of Green Smoothies

1. Green smoothies are very nutritious. I recommend starting with about 60% ripe organic fruit mixed with about 40% organic greens and slowly changing towards 60% greens and 40% fruit.

2. Green smoothies are easy to digest. When blended well, most of the cell walls in the greens and fruits are ruptured, making the valuable nutrients easy for the body to assimilate. Green smoothies literally start to get absorbed in your mouth.

3. Green smoothies, as opposed to juices, are a complete food because they still have fiber. Consuming fiber is important for elimination via the gastrointestinal tract.

4. Green smoothies are among the most palatable dishes for humans of all ages. Fruit taste dominates the flavor, yet the greens balance out the sweetness of the fruit and add a nice zest. People who eat a standard American diet enjoy the taste of green smoothies. They are usually quite surprised that something so green can taste so nice.

5. Green smoothies are chlorophyll-rich. A molecule of chlorophyll closely resembles a molecule of human blood. According to teachings of Dr. Ann Wigmore, consuming chlorophyll is like receiving a healthy blood transfusion. Many people do not consume enough greens, even those who stay on a raw-food diet. By drinking two or three cups of green smoothies daily, you will

consume enough greens to nourish your body; and all of the beneficial nutrients will be well absorbed and assimilated.

6. Green smoothies are easy to make and quick to clean up after. In contrast, juicing greens is time-consuming, messy, and expensive. Many people abandon drinking green juices on a regular basis for these reasons. To prepare a pitcher of green smoothie takes less than five minutes, including cleaning.

7. Green smoothies are loved by children of all ages, including babies of six or more months old. Of course, you have to be careful and slowly increase the amount of smoothie so that the infant's or child's body can get used to the high nutrition in liquefied form.

8. When consuming your greens in the form of green smoothies, you are greatly reducing the consumption of oils and salt in your diet.

9. Regular consumption of green smoothies forms a good habit of eating greens. After a few weeks of drinking green smoothies, most people start to crave and enjoy eating more greens. Eating enough greens is often a problem with many people, especially children.

10. While fresh is always best, green smoothies will keep in cool temperatures for up to three days, which can be handy at work and while traveling.

You will find some green smoothie recipes in Part 4 of this book. Start drinking green smoothies and discover the joys and benefits of this delicious and nutritious addition to your menus. You may find many more amazing facts about green smoothies in my other book, *Green for Life* (see Bibliography).

Chapter 4

MODERN SCIENCE STUDIES UN-COOKING

"All truths are easy to understand once they are discovered; the point is to discover them."

—Galileo Galilee

Igor and I have frequent conversations about the indisputable benefits of eating a raw food-based diet, wondering why it is not more popular worldwide. Having spent countless hours in hospitals, we are aware of how many other people suffer from illnesses similar to ours. We want them to learn about our experience.

Being a professional educator and having deep compassion for all who suffer from health problems, I started teaching classes and sharing the testimonial of my family's experience on the raw diet. Many people became interested and tried this way of eating. However, many of my students inquired about the lack of scientific support that raw-food theory offered. I read all the books about this diet that I could find, visited most of the existing raw-food centers in North America, and took raw- and living-food courses whenever possible. For the classes I offered, I desperately needed as much scientific information as possible. However, in the 1990s, scientific information on the benefits of raw food was scarce. What was available consisted mostly of anecdotal and personal observations. In my presentations, I attempted to explain the theory behind the raw-food diet, using logical, rational, and positive examples. Being aware of the millions of people suffering from the same illnesses that we used to have in my family, I was highly motivated to teach others about the benefits of raw food. I attempted to encourage my audience to try a raw-food diet for a little while so they could experience its benefits for themselves. While this approach satisfied some people, many needed scientific proof to be convinced.

Today, worldwide scientific research that supports the benefits of raw foods comes from two main approaches. The first is the discovery of a variety of beneficial nutrients that exist only in fresh fruits, vegetables, greens, nuts, and seeds. The second direction of scientific research in this area is study of the negative effects of thermal applications to food.

I especially appreciate the discovery of "new" valuable elements in fresh produce. One such example is falcarinol, found in raw carrots. In the last decade, scientists have noticed that consuming fresh carrots seems to reduce the intensity of some cancers. However, in several studies when doctors administered vitamin A or carotene to cancer patients it did not lead to any significant improvements. Finally in 2003, Danish scientists isolated falcarinol in raw carrots. They discovered that even such mild heating of carrots as blanching reduced the falcarinol level by half.[1]

Another important nutrient, resveratrol, promises to lengthen life and prevent or treat aging-related diseases. Resveratrol is found in grapes, grape leaves, red wine, and olive oil, as well as some other vegetables. Researchers have found that the molecules of resveratrol activate a family of enzymes responsible for lifespan in different living organisms including humans.

Another example of beneficial nutrients for human health, phytochemicals (or phytonutrients) promote the functions of the immune system, act directly against harmful bacteria and viruses, reduce inflammation, and are associated with the treatment and prevention of cancer, cardiovascular disease, and any other malady affecting the health and well-being of an individual. It is estimated that at least five thousand phytochemicals have been identified, but a large percentage remain unknown. Many phytochemicals give bright colors to fruits and vegetables. For example, lutein makes corn yellow. Lycopene makes tomatoes red. Carotene makes carrots orange. Anthocyanin makes blueberries blue, and so on. There is abundant evidence from epidemiological studies that the phytochemicals in fresh fruits and vegetables can significantly reduce the risk of cancer.[2]

This new data clearly demonstrate the supremacy of the raw vegan diet. In medical journals and on the Internet, there are now many scientific articles available that demonstrate the dangers of cooked foods, particularly when products are cooked at high temperatures. I selected the following statements from various scientific studies conducted at accredited universities. (Emphasis added in statements.)

"There is ample evidence from basic research of compounds in **cooked and processed meats and fish** ... that heterocyclic amines (HCAs) and polycyclic aromatic hydrocarbons (PAHs) **are mutagens and carcinogens.**"[3]

"Acrylamide is formed during **heating of starch-rich foods** to high temperatures while acrylamide levels are undetectable in uncooked foods. Acrylamide is a 'human carcinogen.' ... Analysis has shown that **acrylamide is present in a disturbingly large number of foods, including many regarded as staple foods—** for example, snack chips, taco shells, French fries, baked potatoes, biscuits, bread, and breakfast cereals. Acrylamide in food is a global problem that requires international action."[4]

"Nine of the 11 studies of raw and cooked vegetables showed statistically significant **inverse relationships of [various] cancers with raw vegetables.** ... Possible mechanisms by which cooking affects the relationship between vegetables and cancer risk include changes in availability of some nutrients, destruction of digestive enzymes, and alteration of the structure and digestibility of food."[5]

"**Heating of fats** brings about measurable changes in their chemical and physical characteristics. Heat is applied in processing for food manufacture, such as during hydrogenation of oils, and in frying for meal preparation. Administration of ... concentrates from thermally oxidized fats **produced cellular damage in hearts, livers, and kidneys** of the lab animals."[6]

"**Cooking meats** at high temperatures and for long duration produces heterocyclic amines and other mutagens. These meat-derived mutagenic compounds have been hypothesized to **increase risk of colorectal cancer.** Consumption of mutagens from meats cooked at high temperature may be associated with high risk of distal colon adenoma."[7]

"In the review of the scientific literature on the relationship between vegetable and fruit consumption and risk of cancer, results from 206 human epidemiological studies and 22 animal studies are summarized. The evidence for a protective effect of greater vegetable and fruit consumption is consistent for cancers of the stomach, esophagus, lung, oral cavity and pharynx, endometrium, pancreas, and colon. The types of vegetables or fruit that most often appear to be **protective against cancer are raw vegetables.** ... Substances present in vegetables and fruit that may help protect against cancer, and their mechanisms, are also briefly reviewed; these include dithiolthiones, isothiocyanates, indole-3-carbinol, allium compounds, isoflavones, protease inhibitors, saponins, phytosterols, inositol hexaphosphate, vitamin C, D-limonene, lutein, folic acid, beta carotene, lycopene, selenium, vitamin E, flavonoids, and dietary fiber. Current U.S. vegetable and fruit intake, which averages about 3.4 servings per day, is discussed, as are effects of increased vegetable and fruit consumption for the benefits against cardiovascular disease, diabetes, stroke, obesity, diverticulosis, and cataracts. **Dietitians are suggested to recommend increasing vegetable and fruit intake in counseling persons."**[8]

"Dietary surveys carried out in the U.S. population indicate that **less than 12 percent of U.S. children and adults meet the recommended level of intake [of vitamin C]. Diet appears to be an important cofactor in the development of obstructive lung disease ... and asthma ...** [New] research should focus on the equally challenging policy issues—namely, **finding effective methods of convincing people to increase their daily consumption of fresh fruits and vegetables."**[9]

"A group of scientists conducted a prospective cohort study of 3,718 participants, aged 65 years and older of the Chicago Health and Aging Project. On measures of mental sharpness, **older people who ate more than two servings of vegetables daily appeared about five years younger** at the end of the six-year study than

those who ate few or no vegetables. Green leafy vegetables including spinach, kale, and collards appeared to be the most beneficial."[10]

Besides acrylamide, HCAs, PAHs, and other mutagens and carcinogens, scientists have discovered yet another large group of
**particularly harmful substances in common foods, resulting from
heating.** In the process of cooking, glucose binds to proteins and
forms abnormally tight (glycated) complexes. They are called
advanced glycoxidation end products (AGEs). These processes are also
known as the Mallard reactions. AGEs have a pathological structure, in which sugars and amino acids are strongly bound together
in an **irreversible connection.** It has been suggested that no other
molecule has the versatility of structure and the potential toxic effects
on proteins as AGEs. Recently, human studies confirmed that about
10% of AGEs consumed with food get absorbed by the body.[11]

AGEs cause cross-linking reactions in blood vessels, in heart
muscle, and in the lens of the eye and thus progressively damage
tissue elasticity. All the muscles in the body, including the heart,
become stiffer. The formation of AGEs and AGE-crosslinks are non-
enzymatic processes and *cannot be reversed* by enzymes that are able
to disrupt other protein bonds. The AGE molecules destroy normal
protein structures, inhibit protein physiologic function, and cause
damage that leads to irreversible disease conditions in vital organs.
AGEs trigger inflammation, especially in patients with diabetes,
neurodegeneration, cardiovascular disease, and kidney failure.[12]

Age-related cardiovascular disorders that are linked to AGEs
include arteriosclerosis, hypertension, stroke, heart failure, and
decreased resilience and flexibility in tendons and ligaments. People with diabetes show substantially larger amounts of AGEs formed

inside the body, due to the high levels of blood glucose. This is why arteriosclerosis, hypertension, stroke, and heart failure are frequent complications in diabetes. In fact, it has been suggested that diabetes is an accelerated form of aging.[13]

You might be surprised to learn that most of us are seeing AGEs every day. AGEs are responsible for the color, flavor, and texture in cooking; they toughen and discolor food—for example, turning a roasting turkey golden brown or darkening a slice of toast. The AGEs could be noted as yellow-brown pigments in the lens of some people's eyes. Due to buildup of AGEs, human lens crystallines become progressively pigmented over time with yellow-brown coloration.[14] Significant accumulation of AGEs may result in liver (age) spots, the brown spots that predominantly occur on sun-exposed areas of the skin and are associated with the appearance of aging.[15]

There is a direct association between dietary AGE intake and a more rapid aging process. The more AGEs we absorb from our food, the more damage we will incur on our biological health. The division of Experimental Diabetes and Aging in the Department of Geriatrics at the Mount Sinai School of Medicine in New York tested 250 foods for their AGE content. The amount of AGEs present in all food categories was related to cooking temperature, length of cooking time, and presence of moisture. Broiling and frying resulted in the highest increased levels of AGEs, while boiling had the lowest. As you will see from Table 1, the amount of AGEs in most fresh foods is relatively small. Huge amounts of AGEs are formed at high temperatures.

The results of this study indicate that cooked food can be a significant dietary source of AGEs, which may constitute a chronic risk factor for cardiovascular problems, kidney damage, and other diseases.[16] The original research document is extensive and contains characteristics of 250 various foods prepared with several different cooking options. To provide examples of some interesting data, I picked a couple of foods from each category for the table below:

Table 1. Advanced Glycoxidation End Products (AGE) Content of Selected Foods

Name of food	Serving (g/ml)	AGE/serving (kU/per serving)
Apple, raw	100	13
Apple, baked	100	45
Banana	100	9
Cantaloupe	100	20
Tomato, raw	100	23
Orange juice, freshly squeezed	250	1
Orange juice, carton	250	14
Avocado	30	473
Butter	5	1,324
Cream cheese, Philadelphia	30	3,265
Peanut butter, smooth	30	2,255
Mayonnaise	5	470
Beef, frankfurter, boiled 7 min	90	6,736
Beef, frankfurter, broiled 5 min	90	10,243
Chicken breast, skinless, raw	90	692
Chicken breast, skinless, boiled 1 hour	90	1,011
Chicken breast, skinless, fried 8 min	90	6,651
Trout, raw	90	705
Trout, roasted 25 min	90	1,924
Cheese, Parmesan, grated	15	2,535

Name of food	Serving (g/ml)	AGE/serving (kU/per serving)
Tofu, raw	90	709
Tofu, sautéed	90	3,447
Cream of Wheat, instant	175	189
Pasta, cooked 8 min	100	112
Pasta, cooked 12 min	100	245
Macaroni and cheese, baked	100	4,070
White potato, boiled, 25 min	100	17
White potato, French fries, homemade	100	694
White potato, French fries, fast food	100	1,522
Lay's Potato Chips	30	865
Chips Ahoy Chocolate Chip Cookies	30	505
Oatmeal raisin cookie	30	411
Club and Cheddar Sandwich Crackers	30	549
Cocoa packet	250	656
Milk, whole	250	12
Milk, fat free	250	1
Milk, fat free, microwave, 1 min	250	5
Milk, fat free, microwave, 2 min	250	19
Milk, fat free, microwave, 3 min	250	86
Formula, infant	30	146
Human milk, fresh	30	2
Pizza, thin crust	100	6,825
Sandwich, toasted cheese	100	4,333

This valuable study demonstrates the destructive power of cooking, especially at high temperatures, and how the destruction drastically increases with each additional minute of heating. Cooking at high temperatures adds to our food a significant amount of AGEs, harmful substances that speed our aging process and can make us ill.

The scientists who study AGEs state in their research papers that formation of AGEs and AGE-crosslinks is normally irreversible. However, based on my own experience and observation, I believe that AGEs and their crosslinks can be reversed—at least partially—by increasing a proportion of fresh fruits and vegetables and reducing consumption of fat in one's diet. I have personally met people who demonstrated to me that their liver spots significantly decreased after several months of consuming predominantly raw food. On the other hand, restriction of cooking time and temperature of cooking food in the diet of patients in another study markedly reduced circulating AGE levels and significantly slowed down a progression of arteriosclerosis, diabetes, and kidney failure.[17]

I predict that for many of my readers, all these strongly negative facts about cooking may come as a surprise, or even a shock. Really, how could a practice so commonly accepted as cooking one's food be harmful? What exactly is happening inside our food when we boil, steam, fry, or roast it?

It is important to understand that, whether we bake a fancy apple pie or merely boil an egg for a few minutes, our food preparation process involves *an application of heat to the food*. From chemistry we know that heat applied to matter causes *endothermic chemical reactions*. All chemical reactions involve the formation or destruction of bonds between atoms. That means that in the process of cooking, the molecules in food gain or lose atoms and become totally different molecules. For example, fresh yams are rich in vitamins A, C, E, K, and B_6, as well as calcium, phosphorus, sodium, magnesium, proteins, and carbohydrates.

These nutrients are extremely beneficial for the human body. How does cooking affect the nutritional content of yams? According to Dr. Gabriel Cousens,[18] cooking makes 50% of the protein unavailable; it destroys 60–70% of the vitamins; and it dramatically reduces other healthy nutrients. In place of the destroyed nutrients, we will most likely find acrylamide, AGEs, and other substances that may cause a wide array of degenerative diseases.

Scientists throughout the world have become alarmed by the latest discoveries about cooking. In 2003, Professor Vincenzo Fogliano of Italy proposed the start of an all-European research on the implications that cooking might have on human health. Twenty-seven European countries signed the memorandum: "Thermally Processed Foods: Possible Health Implications."[19] The participating countries contributed thirty million euros to the foundation for this research, which is now being conducted in numerous European universities simultaneously.

Chapter 5

WHAT IS LIFE?

"Where there is love there is life."

—Mahatma Gandhi

What is the most important ingredient in the human diet? Is it protein? Carbohydrates? Fat? Vitamins? Minerals? All of these components are essential, but I consider the most important element in human food to be *life.* Does cooking our foods add more life to our meals? Unfortunately, the opposite is true: cooking irreversibly destroys the life in our foods.

To illustrate, let us compare two almond seeds (nuts). One seed is raw and one is roasted. To the eye, they look identical; and many nutritionists will claim that they have the same nutritional content. Yet let us put these two seeds in good fertile soil and wait. The one that is roasted will quickly rot, while the raw almond seed will not. The wise little raw kernel will manage to stay intact until springtime. When the waters from melted snow unlock the inhibitors, the almond seed will start to grow into a beautiful tree that will yield thousands more almonds every year. Nothing will ever grow out of the roasted seed.

Obviously, there is a big difference between the raw almond and the roasted one. This difference is as significant as the difference between *life* and *death.* Imagine that somewhere in your body, you need a certain nutrient. Would you want this nutrient to come from an almond that has no life in it, or from the one in which every cell is filled with life?

Every one of us is alive. We think we know a lot about life. Yet do we know exactly *what life is*? This question is more than just complicated: it is, indeed, unanswerable. That's right, to this day, a universal definition of "life" has not been found. Most researchers generally accept that "life is the characteristic state of organisms that exhibit the following common properties:

- they are cellular;
- they are carbon- and water-based with a complex organization;
- they have a metabolism;
- they have the capacity to grow;
- they respond to stimuli;
- they reproduce;
- they adapt through natural selection.

An entity with the above properties is considered to be alive."[1]

I trust that this definition is accurate according to the scientific point of view. However, to me, life is a lot more exciting than merely being an entity that responds to stimuli and has the capacity to grow. Here is my personal perception of the meaning of the word "life."

How do I know that I am alive? It is not because I am moving, since cars are moving too, although they are not alive. It is not because I am breathing, as a vacuum cleaner "breathes" also. It is not because I smile; there are smiling toys in every toy store. I believe that the question "What is life?" is a mystical question, and that life cannot be measured by any scientific means.

I feel my own aliveness through the feelings that come from within me. I feel my own presence inside my body. I feel that I am the life in my body. I care for that life more than for my body itself because I won't care much for my own body after my life ends. I only value my body while my life is in it.

The second "simple" question is, "*Where* is life in my body?" Is it just in my head, or in my heart, or in my fingers, or in the parts that are moving? I feel that life is everywhere in my body, in every one of my 75 trillion tiny cells.

I can see life pouring from people's eyes. They say that eyes are the "windows of the soul." Why do we feel a certain discomfort when looking into another person's eyes? I can look into a doll's eyes and I won't feel any discomfort whatsoever. But when I look into a person's eyes, I definitely experience a sensation, which can sometimes be dramatic. I know that I can sense a lot with my eyes. For example, I can tell if a person is looking at me or not from a remote distance, such as the other side of a soccer field. Many times I have wondered, how am I able to tell? The pupils of the human eye are as tiny as letters in a book. While I cannot read a book from the other side of a soccer field, I can tell for sure if my friend is looking at me because I can feel the connection with this person through our eyes. Awareness of this magnificent power in me, called "life," fills me with joy and appreciation.

There is life in every single cell of the body and maybe even beyond the body. Once, my husband and I participated in a health expo in Canada. Soon after our arrival we discovered the "Advanced Photography" booth that offered pictures of whole-body electromagnetic fields taken with a special camera. Both Igor and I ordered these pictures. We were amazed to discover that our energy on those pictures appeared to be a lot bigger than our physical bodies, and it looked like an oval-shaped cloud. After spending two long, hard-working days at that expo, each one of us took a second picture from the same photographer. This time, we were disappointed because our energy clouds looked a lot smaller and were not evenly shaped. From that experience, I concluded that our life energy is constantly changing, depending on our actions and the conditions in which we live.

From biology, we know that inside plant cells, tiny organelles called "mitochondria" break down carbohydrate and sugar molecules to provide energy. These organelles are alive and constantly at work, but only while the plant is alive, not after it is cooked. Therefore, consuming food that has life in it holds an immense benefit for humans. I have heard from many people that when they stopped eating cooked food, the very first change they noticed was a dramatic increase in their energy levels.

Wild animals intuitively prefer fresher, more alive foods. If given a choice, goats, rabbits, and horses will always choose green grass over hay. We can find numerous examples in nature of various creatures that sustain themselves by eating live food only. For example, a caterpillar from Maui feeds solely on live snails. Most spiders consume exclusively live flies and bugs and would never eat dead insects. If you have ever possessed a lizard as your pet, you know that lizards would rather die from hunger than eat a dead bug, even a freshly caught one. A cheetah eats only fresh meat, consuming just enough to satisfy its hunger.

Of course, there are some animals like vultures, flies, or other scavengers that eat rotten food, including dead meat. However, even those animals do not cook their food. They still get life from their meal but in a different form—as microorganisms. Their bodies have adjusted to digesting decaying food. These creatures usually have a particularly or extraordinarily high concentration of stomach acid capable of killing pathogenic bacteria.

Wild creatures that eat their natural foods rarely develop degenerative diseases. In contrast, it has become almost expected for domesticated animals to develop cancer, diabetes, arthritis, and other illnesses typical of humans who eat the standard American diet. A growing number of vets contend that processed pet food is the main cause of illness and premature death in the modern dog and cat. In December 1995, the *British Journal of Small Animal Practice* published a paper stating that processed pet food suppresses the immune system and damages the liver, kidneys, heart, and other organs. This research, initially conducted by Dr. Tom Lonsdale, was replicated by the Australian Veterinary Association, and was proven to be valid.[2]

Dr. Gyorgy Kollath of the Karolinska Hospital in Stockholm also headed a study of animals. When young animals were fed cooked and processed foods, they initially appeared to be healthy. However, as the animals reached adulthood, they began to age more quickly than normal and also developed chronic degenerative disease symptoms. Members of a control group of animals raised on raw foods aged less quickly and were free of degenerative disease. In nature, we see that wild animals eating entirely enzyme-rich raw foods are free of the degenerative diseases that afflict humans.[3]

I believe the time has come to finally recognize the *most* important ingredient in our food—life, this invisible yet precious quality—and its significance in the realm of health.

Chapter 6

YOUR BODY NEVER MAKES MISTAKES

"Our own physical body possesses a wisdom which we who inhabit the body lack. We give it orders which make no sense."

—Henry Miller

Wouldn't it be nice if every time your car broke down, it would fix itself? This sounds like a fantasy; however, this is just what your beautiful body can do! When you get a cut, the blood washes the dirt out and seals the wound; the skin begins to grow faster; and within a matter of days, you cannot find a trace of injury. If you ingest toxins, your body will develop diarrhea or vomiting to purge the unwanted substance as soon as possible. In the case of injury, our bodies know exactly how to repair themselves in the most efficient way.

Every living thing is dedicated to survival, to prolonging its life to the maximum. Each organism will do its best to adjust to any change in the environment in order to survive. This miracle has been called "The Universal Law of Vital Adjustment." This law has always existed, and it always will. We can see vast evidence of this law in every blade of grass striving to emerge through the concrete, in every rabbit changing the color of its fur with the seasons, and in every human being surviving in today's challenging and constantly changing world. It continues to amaze me how this Universal Law of Vital Adjustment applies to every one of us in many ways. When we understand this important law, we lose the fear that for some mysterious reason our bodies could become ill and that illness could kill us. Our bodies are dedicated to our survival, not our death. The disease-like conditions that our bodies develop, such as coughing, sneezing, fever, pain, and high blood pressure, are in actuality the body's effort to survive. Ironically, when the body heals after taking pills, it most likely heals not because of, but in spite of the medicine. I feel sad that such a serious misunderstanding exists even among many health professionals. I wish scientists would carry out more research on how to help the body heal itself, instead of merely treating its symptoms. By suppressing symptoms, we counteract the wise efforts of the intelligent human body.

According to The Universal Law of Vital Adjustment, our bodies adjust to changes in our environment, including harmful changes such as pollution, radiation, noise, lack of sunlight, etc. Similarly, the body adjusts to the consumption of harmful substances. It develops a new pattern that is actually the best way of coping with the situation. This pattern can quickly become a habit. That doesn't mean that your super-intelligent body is craving harmful substances, but rather that it has adjusted to the toxins. I find it amazing, even amusing, that the human body continues to survive in spite of the many damaging factors of modern life. They include smoking, taking drugs, and overeating harmful foods saturated with chemicals. More and more people spend significant parts of their lifetime indoors without fresh air or sunlight, nearly motionless, surrounded by high-voltage electromagnetic fields and radiation, breathing in all kinds of indoor pollution. They shower daily with fluoridated and chlorinated water, experience constant stress, etc., and on top of that, they adopt numerous smaller habits that may seem innocuous but are in fact additional stressors on the body, like wearing high heels and makeup, sleeping on soft beds, wearing dark glasses, drinking coffee, eating candy, and more. It took me many years to discover that various habits I was lovingly taught to struggle to acquire were actually harmful. In fact, I have changed so many commonly accepted habits that I can't discuss them all in my book, in part for fear of losing credibility. Yet those changes have made my body healthier and my life more joyous.

There is so much confusion in our lives today that we pay top money for workshops and seminars to learn how to do the simplest things that every animal knows naturally. The most popular classes today are not "Is There Life on Mars?" or "How to Become a Millionaire" but those that teach fundamental behaviors, like how to eat, how to sleep, how to run properly, and how to relax. We seek teachers to learn how to stand straight, how to sit correctly, how to see without glasses, how to exercise, and how to spontaneously express emotions. We ask professionals for guidance on issues such as how much water to drink, how to breathe, even how to go to the bathroom. There was a time when we knew all these things naturally. I try to imagine what a natural human being looks like, and I cannot.

Every one of us is living with thousands of adjustments that our body has succumbed to in order for us to survive. We pay for each one of them with reduced quality of health and shortened life span. The way to better health lies in the unburdening of our organisms from having to adjust. However small, every effort towards natural living makes a positive difference. For example, eating more fresh fruits and vegetables, sleeping with an open window at night, wearing clothes made from natural fibers, drinking pure water, exercising, getting sunlight regularly, not suppressing sneezing, yawning, or stretching, and reducing stress can all help. So can turning off electrical devices when not using them to rest from harmful electrical fields, reducing your use of soap and chemicals, buying organic produce, and thousands more small acts, including "applying" a hammer to your microwave oven.

However, one should never introduce new changes into one's lifestyle simply because some authority recommends it. Always observe the reactions your body has to those changes. If you feel better, continue. For example, I used to have a habit of eating before bedtime. When I tried eating just two hours earlier, I immediately began to sleep more soundly. My body showed me that this was a good change, and I adopted this new habit. I realized that such little changes add a great deal of health and enjoyment to my life.

Sometimes our bodies have adjusted to harmful habits so deeply that it takes longer periods of time for the health benefits to surface once the habit is stopped or changed. For example, I used to like to sleep on a soft mattress. Then I read an article describing how healthy it is to sleep on a hard surface. I tried sleeping on the floor but had such an achy back the next morning that I immediately quit. Many years later, I went hiking in the Cascade Mountains and slept on the ground every night for one month. During the first week, I had an achy back. Then my sleep became so sweet, as never before in all my life. Since then I have slept on a hard surface. In addition, soft beds now make my back achy.

I encourage you to follow your own intuition, your own feeling, and your own experience. I do not want you to do anything because somebody who is considered an expert—including me—says so. We are each unique individuals with different bodily requirements. We need to be our own best expert.

Let's do an experiment. If you went to an organic fruit stand today and picked out one fruit, what would it be? A pear, apple, orange, fig, papaya, banana, grape, avocado, mango, or cherry? Do you think that everyone reading this book would pick the same fruit? Most likely not. We are all individuals. Your body knows what you need. Whatever fruit you choose, that is what your body is ordering from you today. Your job is to get your organism what it needs. Tomorrow you may want the same fruit or something new. Let your body lead.

Your body is always ready to act on your behalf. Let's imagine that a piece of dust is falling into your right eye. Which eye will blink? Your right eye, of course. Your left eye won't blink by mistake, because your body never makes mistakes. We have been created perfectly. When we underestimate the wisdom of nature and stop listening to the messages our bodies give us, we get into trouble. Let us take, for example, fever. I trust that if my body has created a fever, then I need a fever. Researchers believe that turning up the heat is the body's way of fighting the pathogens that cause infection by making the body a less comfortable place for them. What is the standard response to fever in our culture? Aspirin. Are we aspirin-deficient? Why do we take aspirin? Aspirin blocks important enzyme activities and can cause gastrointestinal bleeding.[1] Our bodies don't expect this kind of cruelty from us, but they keep fighting for our survival no matter what we do. After we take aspirin, the body immediately re-directs its efforts from the healing process to the removal of aspirin from the organism, because the human body always works on the greater threat first. In the case of taking aspirin, the body is compelled to work especially hard and often becomes so weak that even maintaining a normal body temperature becomes a challenge.

To add insult to injury, when our energy is already low we classically attempt to eat heavy foods, such as chicken soup. However, it's usually the case that when we get ill, we lose our appetite. Our body's message to us is "Don't eat!" And yet we think we need to eat "to have more energy." I used to feed chicken soup to my children when they had a fever. Most of the time they were unable to keep this food down. In response to eating during this "don't eat" stage, a healthy organism attempts to evacuate food from the stomach by throwing up, in order to utilize the maximum amount of energy for healing. Digesting heavy food would severely deplete energy resources that are essential for healing. Cooperating with the body is always the shortest path towards becoming well. Instead of suppressing the fever, we need to help our body conserve energy through eating lighter and resting.

Another example of a useful (if unpleasant) symptom is diarrhea. According to the health research,[2] diarrhea is the body's defense mechanism to minimize contact time between gut pathogens or ingested toxins and intestinal mucosa.

As I write these lines, I become fascinated with the fact that I used to have symptoms such as diarrhea and fever regularly. But since I've adopted a more natural lifestyle, I haven't been sick for many years now. Taking medications to stop fever, diarrhea, or other symptoms works against the wisdom of the body. The body never makes mistakes. If we listen carefully to our bodies, we can all know what we need to do to feel better.

I would like to share with you a story that illustrates how I first began to listen to my body. Some years ago, when my family had been on raw food for only two months, my children began craving different fruits. Sergei asked for mangoes and blueberries, and Valya asked for olives, grapefruits, and figs. When I gave Sergei a mango, he ate it right away and immediately wanted another. As a result, I bought him a whole flat of mangoes, thinking it would last him a week. He ate the entire flat in one day, peels and all. He then said, "I wish there were more mangoes!" The same thing happened with blueberries. I bought him a two-pound bag of blueberries, and he ate it in one sitting.

Valya liked figs. She'd ask for fresh figs, dry figs, black figs, or green figs. She could never have enough figs; she also liked eating olives and grapefruits.

That summer, we visited Dr. Bernard Jensen, a world-famous clinical nutritionist. I asked Dr. Jensen what Sergei needed to eat to help him recover from diabetes. Dr. Jensen looked in his books and told me that the best things for Sergei to eat would be mangoes and blueberries. I was shocked. I then asked him what Valya needed to eat to help her asthma. He said, "Figs, olives, and grapefruits." I couldn't believe his words. I said, "That's exactly what my children have been asking for!" Dr. Jensen then asked me what *my* cravings were. I told him that I didn't know because I always ate what was on sale.

Dr. Jensen helped me to understand that our bodies naturally crave foods that aid healing. My children's bodies communicated with them sooner than my poor confused adult body did. My husband and I started to pay more attention to what our bodies were telling us, and within several weeks, we became aware of our own cravings.

Today, everyone in my family eats slightly differently, even when sitting at the same table. I know that when we develop an appetite for certain *healthy* things (not coffee and doughnuts), it is our bodies asking for particular nutrients.

The human body is more beautiful and wise than we can comprehend. Just remember, *your body never makes mistakes.*

Chapter 7

WHAT THE FIRST HUMANS ATE

"History teaches everything, including the future."

—Alphonse de Lamartine

Once, when I was a little girl, my father took me to an archeological site located near the Azov Sea. There, scientists were excavating the Greek town of Tanais from the fifth century BC. We were surprised to discover that this ancient town was positioned deep in the ground. During the past twenty-five centuries, it gradually became covered by almost thirty feet of dirt. We had to climb down many steps to reach its narrow streets and tiny stone homes surrounded by stone fences. Tanais was so well preserved that it was easy to imagine it full of people. I was mesmerized by my feelings of physical closeness to prehistoric life.

In addition to wandering the streets of Tanais, we were permitted to touch some newly excavated artifacts. Many small, broken, and basically nonessential pieces were left at the site after being thoroughly studied by the scientists. We found many small fragments of ceramic dishes, covered with curious patterns. I especially remember a very unusual-looking petrified fish, which appeared as if it had recently been dried. I immediately made plans to bring this twenty-five-hundred-year-old fish to school with me, but as soon as I touched it with the tips of my fingers, it collapsed into powder.

Not long ago, I found myself equally mesmerized when I read about more recent archeological discoveries. The article talked about the thirteen oldest human skeletons unearthed in East Africa.[1] Scientists dated them at 3.6 million years and named them "the first family." These hominids had curved phalanges, or finger bones, which means that the creatures were agile tree-climbers. They had very thick enamel on their teeth; and their molars were large and square, similar to other creatures that chew lots of greens.[2] Scientists believe that the first humans spent the majority of their time in the branches of trees because that habitat offered much-needed protection from predators and supplied fruit and green leaves; thus the tree-climbing adaptation developed.

These earliest humans, known as Australopithecus, dwelled in East Africa. At that time, the land of East Africa was covered by tropical rainforest. It made sense to me that our ancestors lived in the tropics because heavy annual rainfall, high humidity, and hot temperatures year around ensured an abundance of food. I have heard amazing stories from people who traveled to the tropical rainforest about the countless varieties of fruits—their different shapes, sizes, and colors. Some of these fruits even grow directly off the trunks of the trees. The variety of fruit-bearing plants in the tropical rainforest reaches almost three hundred different species, very few of which have been cultivated.

Sweet fleshy fruits attract not only birds and mammals but also fish, when the fruit rolls into the water. Due to the wealth of fruit, most of the terrestrial animals in the tropical rainforest live in the canopy (the upper part of the trees). There is so much food available up there year around that some animals never descend to explore the forest floor. (I could definitely live like that if only I could get my computer up there!)

Based on my research, I speculate that the food of the first humans *initially* consisted of the following items:

- fruit, due to its abundance and variety;
- green leaves, since many tropical plants are evergreen with broad leaves, the majority of which are edible and exceptionally nutritious;
- blossoms, since most fruit trees develop colorful blossoms that are sweet and nutritious;
- seeds and nuts because they are an important source of protein;
- insects, due to the fact that 90% of the rainforest animal species are insects and most of them are edible and nutritious—a portion of the insects eaten by early humans came directly with the fruit[3]; and
- bark, since tropical trees have exceptionally thin and smooth bark that is often edible and pleasantly flavorful (one example of a popular tropical bark is cinnamon).

Primitive humans were more intelligent than the other inhabitants of tropical forests; therefore, they were capable of harvesting more valuable foods for themselves, leaving less for other species. Since they had more food, they multiplied faster. As the numbers of hominids increased, they inevitably experienced a shortage of food. As plant food became more and more scarce, the primitive humans first increased their consumption of small animals and later began eating larger ones.

The instinctive desire to protect food sources is deeply imprinted in the minds of the vast majority of species on our planet. One may find countless examples of strong territorial behaviors of various creatures in everyday life. Some time ago, I visited a chicken farm in California and was surprised to see that all the birds had the tips of their beaks cut off. The farmers explained to me that whenever chickens don't have adequate space to suit their needs, they begin violently pecking each other—non-stop. I also noticed that despite having no beaks, some chickens were still fighting and many of them were bleeding. I remember watching chickens in my grandmother's yard. They had plenty of space and never pecked each other.

One time I participated in a seminar on the behavior of the wild chimpanzees. The presenter, Hogan Sherrow, had a PhD in Anthropology from Yale University. He described how he lived in the African rainforest and observed the behavioral patterns of these animals. The chimpanzees appeared to be loving and caring creatures in their everyday lives but not when it came to protecting their territory. Approximately once every ten days, the chimpanzee males went on a "walk-about" along the boundaries of their "property" and brutally killed any intruders from other chimpanzee families that they encountered in their territory. I suppose that the first humans were also extremely protective of their territory.

As hominids continued to grow in numbers, their need for food constantly increased. Over the course of three million years, the once-bountiful food sources became scarce; and territories in Eastern and Central Africa became severely overpopulated by hominids. Eventually, they were forced to start moving beyond the rainforest in all directions. By the time of the emergence of *Homo sapiens*, about 120,000 years ago, our forebears were pressured to migrate into the Middle East, South Africa, Europe, Central Asia, and finally into the New World. This migration took many centuries. Researchers estimate that humans migrated to their new territories at a rate of about one mile every eight years.[4]

As humans moved away from the tropics, the most nutritious plant food became more and more scarce and seasonal. Just as all living creatures have the ability to adjust to their environment in order to survive, the bodies of primitive humans began adjusting to the changing climate and food sources available to them. In discussions I often hear speculations on whether primitive people ate meat or not. There can be no doubt that they did. I think every one of us would eat meat if we were faced with similar detrimental circumstances.

In today's life, we occasionally hear survival stories of hikers, skiers, hunters, or rock-climbers who get lost in the woods. From these reports, we learn how those who survived were forced to eat unusual foods, such as bugs, lizards, raw fish, mushrooms, and sometimes even their shoes. Most of these people were only able to last for several weeks. In comparison, two hundred thousand years ago, humans had to survive the long, cold winter months, year after year. They had to go through lengthy periods of hunger, and many of them died from malnutrition. Hominids inevitably tried to consume food of *all* kinds in order to survive. There is no doubt that they tried eating anything that crawled, flew, ran, or swam. Catching birds (along with their eggs), bugs, and other small creatures was a lot easier than catching bigger animals, but small game was not enough to satisfy even one person, let alone an entire tribe. The kill of a big animal could feed a large group for several days. Thus, primitive humans were driven to learn different hunting techniques.

However, early humans were always instinctively drawn back

to eating plant foods whenever they became available because plants, especially greens, are the prime source of human nutrition, as proven by contemporary science.* In addition, plant gathering was not as labor-intensive and dangerous as hunting. Primitive people gathered and consumed a large variety of different plants including greens, fruits, tubers, nuts, seeds, berries, blossoms, mushrooms, sprouts, bark, seaweed, and others. One can only imagine how many different plants they consumed, possibly thousands. In his book *Native American Ethnobotany*, Daniel Moerman, Professor of Anthropology, lists 1,649 species of edible plants that were used by Native Americans alone.[5] That is why we call primitive humans not merely "hunters" but also "gatherers" because indeed hunter-gatherers they were.

To imagine how the first humans discovered grains and eventually bread, I picture myself in the woods two hundred thousand years ago, being cold, scared, barefoot, and hungry, with no food in sight. What would I do? After a futile hunt for some bugs, I would probably search through the dried grasses. Perhaps, there I would find a number of different seeds. I would probably try them and see what they tasted like. I guess that these seeds would be better than nothing at all. But some of them could be awfully hard to chew. If I were smart enough, I would take a stone and try to crush the seeds to make them more edible. If I happened to do it in the rain, eventually I would learn that crushed seeds mixed with water tastes better. I would do this again and again until I invented polenta, bread, porridge, and other pro-bakery foods. For thousands of years, humans ate their "bread" raw. The first bread was nothing but the

---

*Please see Chapter 4 of this book.

crushed seeds of some grasses mixed with water and "baked" on the stones heated by the sun.

Since primitive people had very limited means of preserving plant foods through the cold season, they were forced to hunt more during the long winters. I speculate that most of the meat was eaten by males, while females, who were almost constantly either pregnant or nursing, couldn't hunt very much (nor could small children). If they were not satiated with scraps left by males, females had to seek plant food, even during the wintertime when the plant sources were scarce and less nutritious.

It is an interesting fact that plant cultivation started more than four thousand years earlier than the domestication of animals, even though the process of growing plants was much more complicated than animal training. Early humans did not have rakes and shovels from Ace Hardware, nor did they have the means to irrigate their fields. Collected seeds were extremely hard to protect from rodents and birds. Somehow, early humans managed to plough, sow, weed, water, reap, transport, and so on prior to domesticating animals. In comparison, obtaining a couple of wild baby goats and taming them couldn't have been as difficult.

Nevertheless, the first indications of plant agriculture are found as far back as 11,000 BC, but most likely cultivating of plants started earlier; while animals seem to have been domesticated more than four thousand years later, in 7000 BC.

Thus plant food likely comprised the most essential component of the diet of our ancestors. Through anthropological research, we can see that ancient people valued plant food by how quickly agricultural farming was developed simultaneously in many regions. In 11,000 BC, flint-edged wooden sickles were used to gather wild grains.[6] Eight thousand years ago, wild wheat and barley were grown in ancient Egypt.[7] At the same time, people in Switzerland were growing lentils, and on the island of Crete ancient farmers were growing almonds.[8] Seven thousand years ago, Mesoamericans began growing gourds, peppers, avocados, and amaranths. Five thousand years ago, Chinese people began to cultivate soybeans.[9] They used three hundred sixty-five herbs in their cuisine[10] (which is approximately ten times more than is listed today in the produce section of my local health food store). Four thousand years ago, farmers of Mesopotamia were growing crops of onions, turnips, beans, leeks, lettuce, and garlic.[11]

Plant foods—especially greens—continued to be an important component of the human diet throughout ancient times and into the more recent eras, particularly for economically deprived people. Peasants in villages consumed large amounts of greens. The classical Russian writer, Leo Tolstoi, stated in his book *War and Peace* that "Russian peasants do not get hungry when there is no bread, but when there is no lambsquarters."[12] [Lambsquarters is now considered a weed.—V.B.] Another example can be found in a book by the German poet Johann Wolfgang von Goethe, who observed, "Peasants eat thistle everywhere."[13]

In Russian and Bulgarian languages, the person who sold vegetables was called "zelenschik," which means "the seller of greens." At present time, this word is totally forgotten by people and can be found only in old books and dictionaries. The fact that this word is still listed in dictionaries points to its fairly recent use. From reading classical literature, I know that *zelenschiks* were quite busy only a hundred and fifty years ago, and now they are extinct.

One may find numerous other facts that indirectly point to the popularity of different raw plants in the diet of our ancestors until recent centuries, when the consumption of cooked foods dramatically increased.

For many centuries, humans considered meat to be the healthiest food, probably due to its stimulating taste and lasting satiation. However, the majority of people couldn't afford it and consumed meat only occasionally. People from the upper class dined on a lot of different animal foods—game, fish, beef, pork, sheep, poultry, and eggs almost daily; hence, they were often overweight and suffered from many degenerative ailments. However, even the wealthiest persons consumed large quantities of fruits, vegetables, and greens in various forms, as is illustrated by the following salad recipe from medieval times.[14]

Original Recipe:
Salat. Take persel, sawge, grene garlec, chibolles, letys, leek, spinoches, borage, myntes, prymos, violettes, porrettes, fenel, and toun cressis, rew, rosemarye, purslarye; laue and waishe hem clene. Pike hem. Pluk hem small wip pyn honde, and myng hem wel with rawe oile; lay on vyneger and salt, and serue it forth.

Translation:
Salad. Take parsley, sage, green garlic, scallions, lettuce, leek, spinach, borage, mints, primroses, violets, "porrettes" (green onions, scallions, and young leeks), fennel, and garden cress, rue, rosemary, purslane; rinse and wash them clean. Peel them. [Remove stems, etc.] Tear them into small pieces with your hands, and mix them well with raw oil; lay on vinegar and salt, and serve.[15]

This recipe dates from the fourteenth century and is the earliest such example in English. Most of the recipes were created only for the menus of the upper classes. According to the strict etiquette that ruled medieval mealtimes, the menus included the all-important "order of serving," which meant that most members of a household were entitled to the first course, and the more delicate dishes were served only to the higher ranks. Interestingly, we can see how it was thought natural to eat the most nutritious foods first (salads), leaving the richer and sweeter courses for later.

In addition to fresh fruits and vegetables consumed during the summer by people of the Middle Ages, they stocked a supply of fruits and vegetables in their cellars for the cold seasons. They fermented large quantities of sauerkraut; marinated mushrooms; and pickled tomatoes, cucumbers, carrots, apples, beets, turnips, cranberries, garlic, and even watermelons. Such preserved vegetables were kept in wooden tubs in cellars. Both rich and poor people kept tubers, dried mushrooms, dried herbs, apples, nuts, and dried fruits for the winter. They also prepared a supply of dried fish, meat, and bacon. An important source of vitamins came from the barrels of fermented juices of different fruits, berries, and wines. Most of the food in the cellar was raw.

Chapter 8

CONVENIENCE VERSUS HEALTH

"I would cook dinner, but I can't find the can opener!"

—**Author Unknown**

Our ancestors ate only raw foods for more than three million years. When early humans mastered the use of fire, approximately 790,000 years ago,[1] they didn't start cooking right away. For many thousands of years, ancient people used fire for warmth, light, and safety from predators. It is logical to suggest that they did not start using fire for cooking on a regular basis until the very end of the hunter-gatherer period because they couldn't possibly carry fire with them or start a new fire from scratch every day. Moreover, hunter-gatherers couldn't carry much of anything with them including food for evening cooking—because all they had were their bodies. Early humans had to be ready to run or climb at any moment. Carrying meat would be particularly dangerous because it could attract hungry predators to the tribe.

Starting a new fire, especially in adverse weather, requires a great deal of time and labor. I tried starting fire by friction many times during hikes with my family, and just igniting the kindling took half an hour or more. Then one needs to build up flames big enough for cooking, which in turn takes another hour or two. I imagine that early humans were feeding throughout the day as they found food, rather than having cooked lunches or dinners. I speculate that even when they settled and started living in permanent places, eating cooked food was still a rare occurrence until the invention of the stone hearth oven in 5000 BC.

Even then, cooking continued to be a luxury for many centuries due to the labor involved and the effort needed to acquire firewood, which was the sole fuel used for millennia. Today it is hard to believe that housewives and cooks had to start the fire in their hearth by the use of either sparking flints or friction methods until 1827, when English chemist John Walker invented matches. Considering all these obstacles, it is not surprising that cooked food was the most expensive and thus considered the more valuable food.

Ancient people (like many moderns!) were not aware of the components of proper nutrition. They believed the most delicious and stimulating foods to be the healthiest. Throughout the history of humankind, some genius minds such as Anaxagoras, Hippocrates, and Leonardo da Vinci conveyed their brilliant theories but were not taken seriously by the majority of people.

For thousands of years, while early humans ate predominantly raw food, they were making their food choices solely by applying their instincts, which kept their diet as nutritious as possible. That was why they were able to survive through millions of years, despite all the famine, predators, and drastic climate changes.

We now know that the process of cooking is a chemical reaction that alters the components in food. As a result, cooking produces toxic molecules that can act as stimulants and create false cravings. When humans increased their consumption of cooked food, they followed their bodily cravings and not their instincts. As a result, humans slowly became increasingly malnourished. Certain groups of people who sustained themselves mostly on cooked or processed products developed such severe diseases as scurvy, rickets, beriberi, and pellagra. These ailments took many thousands of human lives year after year until relatively recently. For example, in 1915, more than ten thousand people died of pellagra in the United States alone.[2]

While throughout most of human history, the majority of people have eaten primarily raw plant foods, with the development of civilization, this pattern quickly began to change. The most dramatic increase in consumption of cooked and highly processed foods occurred quite recently, during the very end of the eighteenth and the beginning of the nineteenth centuries, when three major industrial developments took place almost simultaneously.

- In the late eighteenth century, a Swiss miller invented a steel roller mechanism that simplified the grinding process and led to the mass production of white flour. In 1784, American inventor Oliver Evans developed the first automated flourmill.[3]
- In 1813, British chemist Edward Charles Howard invented a method of refining sugar.[4]
- In the nineteenth century, the process of canning started. It was Napoleon who announced a competition for the best way of preserving food for his army. In 1795, French chef Nicholas Appert won the prize of 12,000 francs for inventing a method of canning meats and vegetables in jars sealed with pitch. For a while, it was a French military secret but soon it leaked across the English Channel. In 1810, Peter Durance, an Englishman, patented the use of metal containers for canning; and one year later, there were several canning factories in operation. The troops that faced off at Waterloo had canned rations.

The demand for canned food was so great that canning technology began developing quickly; and by the 1860s, the time it took to process food in a can had been reduced from six hours to thirty minutes.[5] Canned foods were soon commonplace. Tin-coated steel is still used today. All canned foods were thoroughly cooked; preservatives and salt were added to enhance shelf life. Typically, canned products have a shelf life of a good two years or more.

These inventions were embraced by everyone—by people who appreciated the convenience and lesser costs, by merchants for the chance to make more profits, and by the governments for an opportunity to provide cheaper food to people. In the course of the nineteenth century, the majority of people in civilized countries began to consume a drastically larger percentage of highly processed foods, and, accordingly, lowered their percentage intake of nutritionally dense foods.

I appreciate many wonderful and brilliant discoveries made by humanity during the years of the Industrial Revolution. Yet, the radical transformation of the human diet was rather destructive. Lifesaving habits and instincts practiced by the collective effort of millions of previous generations were lost in virtually no time. While the human body was still the same, the food was quickly and severely changed.

Meanwhile, devitalized foods in shiny cans, puffy white breads, and various confections were not only appreciated for their low costs and high convenience but became a symbol of human progress. These new products liberated women from hours of cooking every day and even from nursing their infants. For the first time in human history, babies were fed with formula, which was considered equally fine or even superior to breast milk. Nearly all foods for adults turned into formula, too. In place of naturally nutritious products, people now consumed a large assortment of canned foods, which they opened with a special device (can opener), accompanied by wide selection of cheeses and sausages on slices of snow-white bread, concluding their meals with an ever-growing amount of candy, wrapped in fancy foils.

It is no surprise that at the same time cancer death rates and incidents of other degenerative diseases started to explode. By the year 1900, 64 people out of 100,000 died from cancer. These already high numbers continued to grow and in fact tripled by the year 2000.[6] In the United States during the last few years, cancer surpassed heart disease and became the number-one cause of death. The American Cancer Society estimated that 1,399,790 men and women would be diagnosed with cancer, and 564,830 men and women would die of cancer of all types in 2006.[7]

In the twentieth century, nutrition began to emerge as a science simultaneously in several countries. With the formulation of the general concept of vitamins in 1912[8] and discovery of vitamin C in 1931, scientists started conducting more research on the human diet. During the first part of the twentieth century, public nutrition programs generally recommended increasing the consumption of practically everything in the usual diet, applying the idea that "excess is preferable to limitation."[9] The surprise came "during the second world war, when supplies of food and particularly of animal foods in European countries were severely restricted, [and] the incidence of some diseases was generally reduced."[10]

The science of nutrition is very young, less than a century old, but it is developing rapidly. Almost daily we hear of discoveries of totally new (to us), yet vitally necessary nutrients. For centuries, humans didn't know which components of diet were the most essential for their health. Many people considered tasty foods to be the healthiest. Such ignorance has taken scores of lives. At the same time, a properly balanced diet can ensure optimal health performance for all people. Yet we consume tons of highly processed foods today, more than ever before in human history. What is even more alarming is that we love our processed foods to such an extent that we prefer them to natural products. This causes a dependency on cooked food. I believe that our ability to end this dependency can change the future of humankind.

Chapter 9

HOW MY FAMILY EATS

"In this plate of food, I see the entire universe supporting my existence."

—A Zen blessing at mealtime

Is it expensive to stay on raw food? Yes and no. Let me explain. In order to be understood correctly, I am going to pull out my receipts and share in detail exactly what I spend. For my family of four, I spend on average $45 per day. That comes to $1,350 per month; but if divided by four, it is only $338 per person. I would like to clarify that we spend this much money on food not because we are very rich, but because we do not have health insurance; and we consider our health to be the priority among all of our expenses. My intent is to *not* save money when it comes to nourishing the body. I am aware that I need to receive adequate nourishment not only for today's performance but also to make up for thousands of days in the past when my body was malnourished. I would rather reduce spending on other things: furniture, clothing, household chemicals, fancy cars, and surely health insurance.

There were times when my family didn't have much money. Once, for two years, the four of us lived on a total budget of $900 per month. That included car insurance, gas, and the rest of our expenses. My children like to remember the Christmas of 1997 when Valya received a hair band for a present, and Sergei got a pencil. For some reason, they cherish the memory of that holiday more than any other. Even then, we managed staying on a high-quality raw-food diet. We discovered many different ways of obtaining good produce for little money or at no cost at all; we just had to spend more of our time sorting or gathering produce rather than buying it. Igor built a special attachment to our van for growing sprouts in jars, in two large coolers. We constantly had an abundance of fresh sprouts for the cost of pennies. We approached different organic farmers and offered our help in exchange for fresh fruits and vegetables. We bought marked-down organic produce from the health food stores. We learned to arrive at farmers' markets at the end of the day to get the best deals on their goods. By attending several wild walks with experts, we acquired foraging skills and started gathering wild edibles during most of the year. We went to countless U-picks and gathered anything from cucumbers to peaches. Finally, we offered help in picking fruit to owners of fruit trees who did not have time for harvesting. Many times people were curious about what we were going to do with so much fruit and were quite surprised that we considered persimmons or cherries to be an important part of our diet. We ran into families that lived in big mansions but who ate very poorly. We were poor, but we sure ate like kings and queens, or I should say, as "educated kings and queens."

Today all four of us work and we are happy to be able to buy all our food from health food stores and farmers. I am committed to obtaining only the best-quality, fresh organic produce, preferably seasonal and locally grown. During the warm seasons of the year, we buy most of our produce from farmers. I love talking to organic farmers. I consider them all to be heroes for their dedication to natural gardening despite tremendous challenges and hard labor involved.

I am fortunate to have a health food store two blocks from my house that I visit every other day (or three to four times a week) to buy food for my family. My husband and children like to help, but I do most of the food shopping. Typically, I bring with me several cloth bags that I fill with produce. In the wintertime, I alternate buying a case of apples or pears every week, to always have fresh organic fruit on hand at the house. Buying in bulk saves me twenty percent of the retail cost.

When I began consuming green smoothies and was looking for ways to increase the variety of greens, I went to the growers' market and spoke to at least ten farmers. I offered to pay each one of them $20 for bringing me a large box of edible weeds the following week. I believe that wild edibles are our true superfood. Two farmers became interested. Both of them have been bringing me chickweed, stinging nettles, lambsquarters, thistle, plantain, dandelions, purslane, and many other different edible greens on a weekly basis since then. Because of this supply of the most nutritious greens, I stopped buying greens from the store almost completely from April to October. Encouraged by my support, these farmers offered edible weeds to our local co-op; and I was pleased to see these most nutritious greens there for sale.

During the rest of the year, I usually buy eight bunches (two days' worth) of different greens from the store, including but not limited to the following: dandelion, kale, chard, spinach, romaine, cilantro, parsley, scallions, collard, arugula, frisee, escarole, and endive. Once a week I purchase a bag of baby greens mix. For two days' consumption for my family, I usually buy twelve avocados, eight ripe, bright yellow lemons, and a bunch of bananas.

I consider that the fruit variety is not perfect in any of the stores because most of the fruit has been picked unripe. I also find it frustrating that I cannot enjoy seeded grapes anymore. I always buy the fruit that is the ripest of all, and sometimes I ask the produce manager if he has riper fruit in the back. Typically I buy one pound each of three to four different fruits, such as mangoes, pineapples, papayas, grapefruits, kiwis, figs, persimmons, or whatever is in season. I always buy a lot of berries, as they are less hybridized, riper than other fruit, and rich in many essential nutrients. I usually buy four to five pints of different berries. I almost never buy watermelon, except when it is in season, because I only buy the best organic seeded watermelons directly from farmers.

I usually buy a dozen ripe tomatoes, two to three firm cucumbers, and a couple of red or yellow bell peppers. I never buy green bell peppers, as they are unripe. Once or twice per month, I buy several carrots or beets to shred them in our salad. Approximately once a month, I buy a bag of dates, choosing a different brand each time.

About every other month, I place a bulk order for a five-pound bag of sunflower seeds, a five-pound bag of almonds, a two-pound bag of chia seeds, and a twenty-five-pound bag of flax seed (that might seem like a lot, but we share a large portion of our flaxseed crackers with friends).

I do not buy chocolate or raw cacao beans. I also do not buy any kind of salt but only sea vegetables: kelp, dulse, nori, arame, and others. I do not buy oil, as we stopped using oils altogether a while ago. However, I cannot guarantee that we will stay away from oils forever. In my family, we are following our intuitive guidance rather than other people's recommendations. We attempt to consume fats in a more natural form rather than using oil—for example coconuts, avocados, occasional durians, and a small amount of seeds and nuts. I especially enjoy sea buckhorn berries that I pick in August through September in a local garden. I consider sea buckhorn berries to be a wonderful source of healthy oils, folic acid, B-vitamins, and many other important nutrients.

Often people ask my family to describe what we eat in the course of a day. I will tell here what I eat.

I always have one quart of green smoothie for breakfast, around 8 a.m. If I remember, I snack on a piece of fruit around noon. In other cases, I get so busy with work, which I love, that I forget about my snack.

We have a tradition, almost a ceremony, to eat green soup with our friends and family every day at two o'clock in the afternoon. Whether at my office or at home, one of us quickly prepares green soup, which consists of just four ingredients, in a Vita-Mix blender. This soup is incredibly satisfying, and it is the most essential meal of my day.

When I come home at 7 p.m., I have another smoothie accompanied by either a bowl of greens and veggies without any dressing, or a bowl of fruit. Another option for my dinner is a bowl containing a pint of berries topped with a spoonful of raw almond butter, which we grind ourselves. I really would like to not eat anything else, but I do eat an apple or two later in the evening.

I am providing this information only as a means of sharing and not as recommendation. Please do not try to copy me—keep in mind that it took me more than twelve years to come to this way of eating, and it is continuously changing. Follow your inner guidance and treat yourselves as if you were well-educated kings and queens.

Chapter 10

BACTERIA—NATURE'S BRILLIANT INVENTION

"It is about time we take a closer look at the Bacterial Kingdom, with capitals. For a Kingdom it is, biologically speaking, and the ancient lineage, diversity, and evolutionary power of its inhabitants deserve royal treatment rather than disgust."

—Trudy Wassenaar, PhD, a molecular biologist

I want to share my amusement with and appreciation for bacteria. Maybe your respect for them will grow after reading this chapter. Bacteria are the world's greatest recyclers. By transforming all dead organic matter into soil, bacteria recycle useless garbage into the source of all elements. Bacteria are unique; they are tiny and huge at the same time. Smaller than any living cell, bacteria can instantly increase their power by multiplying into "zillions" more. Each bacterium is capable of producing 16 million more in just 24 hours.[1] Therefore, whether bacteria need to decompose ten dead elephants or one dead ant, bacteria will always have plenty in their army; and no rotting will be delayed due to the lack of little critters. Bacteria are nature's brilliant invention and gift to us all. We are constantly trying to destroy as many bacteria as possible because we don't understand their purposes on Earth. Let us imagine life without bacteria. There would be rocks but no soil in which to grow food. All dead trees, animals, birds, insects, snakes, human bodies, or other organic matter would be piled into huge mountains. What a mass of clutter that would be!

Perhaps you have noticed that in a natural setting, bacteria in the rotting cycle do not cause an offensive odor. In the forest, nobody rakes the leaves or buries the animals; everything is just left in the open. The droppings of animals and birds are left where they've fallen. You would expect the forest to smell bad. Yet the last time you were in the forest, did it smell bad? I bet your answer is "no." In fact, when we go to the forest, we breathe in and say, "Ah, it smells so good!" If bacteria don't produce smell in the natural habitat of the forest, then why do we associate rotting with odor?

Healthy soil contains a large percentage of "good" bacteria. Friendly bacteria manufacture many essential nutrients for the plants that grow in this soil. Such "good" or aerobic bacteria flourish in the presence of oxygen and require it for their continued growth and existence. "Good" bacteria thrive in the soil with a large amount of organic matter, such as parts of plants and dead animals. When there is a lack of oxygen or organic matter in the soil, "bad" bacteria take over and begin to multiply, causing an extremely offensive odor. These pathogenic bacteria are anaerobic and cannot tolerate gaseous oxygen. While pathogenic bacteria create offensive odors and may cause disease, they serve their own imperative purpose. That is why in nature there is a balance of "good" and "bad" bacteria, with a significant dominance of "good" bacteria. "Good" bacteria can be easily destroyed by countless factors, such as chemical fertilizers and pesticides in soil, and in the human body by antibiotics, a poor diet, overeating, stress, etc.

That is why, in the civilized world, bacteria create foul smell.

Bacteria have a hard time decomposing the unnatural substances we create. To test this statement, you may conduct your own experiment. Put raw fruits and vegetable scraps into your compost. You will notice that they will rot and disintegrate without a bad odor. Now add to your compost some cooked food such as cooked noodles, chicken soup, or mashed potatoes. After a few days, you will notice an unpleasant odor emanating from your compost. The smell could be so bad that your neighbors might complain.

Bacteria play a major role in growing nutritious produce. The main difference between organic and conventional gardening is that "Conventional agriculture attempts to feed the plants while the organic method nourishes the microorganisms in soil."[2] In simple words, conventional farmers ignore the microorganisms in the soil and aim their efforts at supplying potassium, nitrogen, and other chemicals for the sake of plants, while organic gardeners take care of feeding the living things in the soil, which provide harmoniously balanced nutrients to the plants. Just as humans cannot live on chemicals instead of food, microorganisms in the soil cannot survive when fed artificial fertilizers only. When all microorganisms get destroyed with chemicals, the soil turns to dust. No plants can grow in dust, no matter how rich in various chemicals this dust is.

Through the plants we eat, we receive essential nutrients that were created by microorganisms in the soil. The more organic matter or "humus" present in the soil, the more nutritious is the food grown in this soil. We humans have inherited many feet of beautiful, fruitful topsoil all around the globe with zillions of happy microorganisms thriving in it. In their best-selling book, *Secrets of the Soil*, Peter Tompkins and Christopher Bird state: "The combined weight of all the microbial cells on Earth is twenty-five times that of its animal life; every acre of well-cultivated land contains up to a half a ton of thriving microorganisms, and a ton of earthworms which can daily excrete a ton of humic castings."[3]

As a result of our "highly technological" gardening, most of the soil at agricultural farms in the USA contains less than 2% organic matter, while originally, before the era of chemistry, this figure was 60–100%. According to David Blume, an ecological biologist, permaculture teacher, and expert, "Most Class-1 commercial agricultural soil is lucky to hit 2% organic matter—the dividing line between a living and dead soil."[4] By applying permaculture gardening techniques to a field of extremely depleted soil, which consisted of cement-hard adobe clay, David Blume was able to bring the organic matter to the 25% level within a couple of years. From this field, he harvested the crops at a rate "8 times what the USDA claimed is possible per square foot."[5]

We cannot successfully feed soils with chemicals because "biology does not equal chemistry."[6] In other words, chemical fertilizers are missing live enzymes, which contribute to the most productive and unique qualities of all soils.

Another interesting fact is that all living things have a strong immunity that doesn't let bacteria enter the body of plant, animal, or human until this organism dies. Bacteria can never disintegrate anything that is still alive. For example, gigantic redwood trees can exceed two thousand years of age, yet they remain free of decay. Their roots are always in the soil, yet bacteria do not touch them. However, as soon as the tree dies, the bacteria move in to return the tree to its source—the soil. Bacteria can tell what is living and what is dead, and they are only interested in dead matter.

We can find many more examples in nature of how different

parasites can attack only plants or animals with a weakened immunity. For instance moss, mistletoe, and lichens don't live on strong, healthy trees. Healthy, balanced soil in organic gardens results in sturdy plants, which deter slugs and insects. Tree mushrooms grow mainly on fallen logs or dying trees in the forest. Similarly, bacteria and parasites don't live off healthy flesh. Since immunity is the *only* existing barrier for parasites, why not put all our efforts into strengthening our immunity, instead of trying to poison bacteria? The same applies to any parasite. If we keep our body clean, healthy, and nourished, parasites cannot live in our body ecology, and even mosquitoes won't bite us.

Maintaining personal hygiene is essential; but at the same time, we are unable to control the presence of all bacteria in every place, no matter how well we clean and how many chemicals we apply. With much effort, strict law, and financial investments, we have now gained almost complete control over spreading bacteria through public bathrooms. There are high-tech hand dryers and sophisticated toilet seat covers. One can go through the entire visit to a public restroom without touching anything. Yet there are still plenty more places where humans could encounter "bad" bacteria that are next to impossible to control. For example: shopping cart handles, car doors, pens at the post office, store, or bank, handrails in the public transportation system, escalators, and elevators, money, serving utensils at all-you-can-eat restaurants, automated bank machines, and many more, including food containers such as cans, buckets, and boxes. In comparison to the enormous task of destroying all "bad" bacteria in our environment, improving bodily immunity seems a lot more sensible and doable.

Ironically, all antibacterial agents that we apply to our bodies destroy not only the "bad" bacteria but also the "good" microorganisms, which are an important part of our natural immunity against "bad" bacteria. I see in this action more damage than worth. To me, it is like cutting a finger off just because it has a splinter in it. Instead, let us be afraid of our cleaning supplies, most of which are poisonous chemicals. Bacteria cannot harm us if we follow the laws of nature, but chemicals eventually *will* kill all of us if we do not drastically reduce their utilization. Therefore, if we are afraid of infectious disease, the best thing we can do is strengthen our immune system through eating nutritious food, exercising, applying stress-reducing techniques, and using other natural ways of healing.

Chapter 11

WHAT ABOUT INSECTS?

"The pure and simple truth is rarely pure and never simple."

—Oscar Wilde

Presently, I am not for or against eating insects. However, I would consider myself an idealist if I didn't address this subject. Furthermore, I have been asked the question about insects at almost all of my lectures. Thus, despite being vegan for many years and feeling a personal repulsion towards the very idea of consuming bugs, I decided to share with you what I have found.

The chief fact to consider is that most, if not all, human groups or tribes throughout our history have consumed insects. Almost all ancient people, including Native Americans, considered insects a wonderful food source. To some, insect food was a matter of survival; to others, a delicacy.[1]

According to a Purdue University study,[2] at present time, 80% of the people in the world consume insects deliberately and on a regular basis; and 100% eat them unintentionally. There are 1,462 recorded species of edible insects. Dishes that include different bugs are served in many gourmet restaurants in Japan, France, Taiwan, Australia, New Zealand, Thailand, and other countries. Edible insects are and have been traditionally an important and nutritious food for people in Africa, Asia, Australia, and Latin America for centuries.[3] The natives of southern Africa have used a number of insects as food, including caterpillars, locusts/grasshoppers, ants, termites, and beetles.[4] Many people consume crawfish, lobster, crab, and shrimp, which are part of the insects' biological phylum—arthropods.

There is much historic evidence of the human consumption of insects throughout history:

- The ancient Romans and Greeks dined on insects. Pliny, the first-century Roman scholar and author of *Historia Naturalis*, wrote that Roman aristocrats loved to eat beetle larvae reared on flour and wine.[5]

- Aristotle, the fourth-century Greek philosopher and scientist, described in his writings the ideal time to harvest cicadas: "The larva of the cicada on attaining full size in the ground becomes a nymph; then it tastes best, before the husk is broken. At first the males are better to eat, but after copulation the females, which are then full of white eggs."[6]

- The Old Testament encouraged Christians and Jews to consume locusts, beetles, and grasshoppers (Leviticus 11:21–23). St. John the Baptist is said to have survived on locusts and honey when he lived in the desert (Matthew 3:4).

Insects are regarded as the most successful group within the animal kingdom. More than 80% of all living animals are insects. About one million species of insects are known; and at least 7,000 new species are discovered and described every year. Prominent reasons for their success are as follows: the ability to live in and adapt to diverse habitats, a high reproductive capacity, the ability to consume different kinds and qualities of food, and the ability to escape quickly from their enemies.[7]

According to William F. Lyon of Ohio State University,

> If Americans could tolerate more insects (bugs) in what they eat, farmers could significantly reduce the amount of pesticides applied each year. It is better to eat more insects and less pesticide residue. If the U.S. Food and Drug Administration would relax the limit for insects and their parts (double the allowance) in food crops, U.S. farmers could apply significantly less pesticides each year. Fifty years ago, it was common for an apple to have worms inside it, bean pods with beetle bites, and cabbage with worm-eaten leaves.

> Most Americans don't realize that they are probably already eating a pound or two of insects each year. One cannot see them, since they have been ground up into tiny pieces in such items as strawberry jam, peanut butter, spaghetti sauce, applesauce, frozen chopped broccoli, etc. Actually, these insect parts make some food products more nutritious.[8]

Professor Lyon speculates that "Many insects are far cleaner than other creatures. For example, grasshoppers and crickets eat fresh, clean, green plants whereas crabs, lobsters, and catfish eat any kind of foul, decomposing material as a scavenger (bottom water feeder). According to the Entomological Society of America, by weight, termites, grasshoppers, caterpillars, weevils, houseflies, and spiders are better sources of protein than beef, chicken, pork, or lamb. Also, insects are low in cholesterol and low in fat."[9]

According to Dr. Joseph Mercola, author of *Total Health Program* and several other popular books: "Many insects have vitamin B_{12} ... for example, five termite species contained large amounts of B_{12}

(.455–3.21 mcg/mcg)."[10] To compare, the USDA daily recommendation of vitamin B_{12} is 2.8 micrograms for adults.[11] This may help explain how primitive humans could have obtained B_{12} without needing to rely on large amounts of meat.

In 2002, twenty people were competing for $50,000 in a reality show, *The Last Hero*. One of their tasks was to eat a bowl of live worms and beetles. In their interviews after the show, the participants shared how they were surprised that they actually liked the taste of those insects and were even looking forward to eating more.

Virtually everything we eat has insects (entire bugs or parts of them) within; indeed, there are government standards as to the maximum number of bug parts per unit for each type of food permitted. U.S. regulations allow for 75 insect fragments per 50 grams of wheat flour, two maggots per 100 g of tomato sauce or pizza, 20 maggots for canned mushrooms, 60 fragments per 100 g of peanut butter, and so on.[12] These levels are set because it is not possible, and never has been possible, to grow in open fields, harvest, and process crops that are totally free of natural defects.

The alternative to establishing natural defect levels in some foods would be to insist on increased utilization of chemical substances to control insects, rodents, and other natural contaminants. The alternative is not satisfactory because of the very real danger of exposing consumers to potential hazards from residues of these chemicals, as opposed to the aesthetically unpleasant but harmless natural and unavoidable defects. "Noting the widespread use of pesticides in industrial agriculture, people are poisoning the planet by ridding it of insects, rather than eating insects and keeping artificial chemicals off plants that we eat."[13]

According to Gene DeFoliart, a professor emeritus of entomology at the University of Wisconsin-Madison, "In our preoccupation with cattle, we have denuded the planet of vegetation. Insects are much more efficient in converting biomass to protein."[14] Insect farming is arguably much more efficient than cattle production. One hundred pounds of feed produces 10 pounds of beef, while the same amount of feed yields 45 pounds of cricket.[15]

I speculate that the prejudice towards insects started in Western countries with the discovery of bacteria. When the public developed fear and disgust for microbes, these emotions were spread onto insects.

Since I have been vegan for many years, I decided to ask my friends whom I regularly meet at our vegan potlucks what they think about eating insects. We had a buzzing discussion with a wide array of opinions. At first everybody said that we should not hurt any other living things at all. However, after going deeper into the subject, my friend Mike came up with some unexpected observations. The following are his main considerations. If humans would consume insects:

- They will be compelled to use less pesticides, and fewer insects will be killed as a final result.
- Consumers would not be afraid of insects in their food, such as fresh produce, pasta, or chocolate, and as a result they could expect less pesticides in their products.
- Non-vegetarian consumers would consume less meat from animals that have nervous systems and which experience profoundly more suffering.
- Organic gardeners, who handpick large volumes of beetles off the plants in vegan gardens, could eat or sell their insects rather than destroying them.

In summary, if people in Western countries will simply *feel more comfortable* around insects, it would benefit many larger animals, help insects on a larger scale, and support ecology in general, apart from any potential benefits to human health.

Part 2

HUMAN DEPENDENCY ON COOKED FOOD

Chapter 12

IS IT REALLY A DEPENDENCY?

"We are slow to believe that which if believed would hurt our feelings."

—Ovid, Roman poet, 43–18 BC

When my family went on a raw-food diet, I was surprised how difficult it was for me to stay on a strict raw regimen, especially during the first two weeks. At first, I thought that my cravings for cooked food were caused simply by my love for home cooking. My longing for cooked cuisine lasted approximately two months, then little by little I forgot about the mere existence of cooked delicacies and I became content with my family's new way of eating. My husband experienced distress similar to mine and it also took him two months to settle into a raw-food diet. Our children's conversion from cooked to raw food seemed to happen much faster and smoother than ours.

Later, when I began teaching raw-food classes, I discovered that transitioning to raw food is not easy for the majority of people. There seemed to be a contradiction. On one hand, there was a lot of interest in learning about the raw-food diet and my classes were full. On the other hand, many of my students revealed to me that staying on a raw-food diet even for one or two days was amazingly challenging for them. The contradictory feedback that I heard over and over again was that people loved how they felt while eating only raw food—energized and youthful, better than ever before—but they couldn't remain on this diet because of strong cravings for cooked food that emerged right away. For instance, I remember two sisters; both of them suffered from hypoglycemia. They were so excited about becoming raw-foodists that they stayed after my lecture and asked me to help them with their raw-food plan. However, the very next day, when I accidentally ran into them at a health food store, the sisters greeted me by nodding while hiding their hands behind their backs. As they were passing, one of them dropped . . . a muffin. Apparently they underestimated the power of those muffins.

In order to explore the effectiveness of my teaching, I conducted a survey among participants of my workshops. I discovered with amusement that in one month after my lectures, only 2% of my students were still eating 80% or more raw food. In disbelief, I conducted another survey, which happened to fall on January, right after the holiday season. Naturally, there were no raw-fooders left among my students at all.

Initially I decided that it was my fault as a teacher and that I should make my nutrition classes more engaging. I tried my best to be a fun teacher. I even sang Russian folk songs in my classes, told hilarious jokes, and shared my best raw-food concoctions with the class. Nonetheless, the outcome was still the same: most people who signed up for my classes enjoyed how they felt on a raw-food diet but were unable to stick to it.

One day, my friend Gerry invited me to his AA (Alcoholics Anonymous) meeting. I'd never been to an AA meeting before and I was deeply touched by the sincerity of people when they spoke about their addictions. At this meeting I was struck by the idea that maybe cooked food is also an addiction. In fact, if cooked food were not an addiction, people would sometimes accidentally miss cooked meals and would live a day or two once in a while totally on raw food. However, that never happens in one's entire life except for the occasions when one is lost in the woods or something similarly dramatic happens. Just as a smoker doesn't miss a day without a cigarette, people who habitually eat cooked food feel a need to consume at least some cooked food daily. No wonder most people believe that cooked food is essential for human health.

After all this reasoning, I went to the library in our town and checked out about thirty books on addiction. The librarians looked at me with pity. They must have thought I had a big problem.

I found a lot of helpful information in those books. I learned that people with an addiction suffer from an irresistible need to use a certain substance despite knowing the serious physical or emotional results. I found out that the three main symptoms of addiction are:

- denial that there is a problem;
- the feeling of needing the substance to function normally;
- overuse of a substance (alcohol, food, tobacco, or other).[1]

These descriptions reminded me of my own remarkably similar relationships with cooked food. Now I understood why my transition to a raw-food lifestyle was so difficult. I realized that my suffering was not caused by eating raw food but by *not eating* cooked food. And my cravings for cooked dishes were nothing but a sign of withdrawal from cooked foods. I now saw why my teaching had not been very effective. I taught only about the benefits of raw food and how to prepare delicious raw recipes, but failed to provide a most needed understanding of the addictive nature of cooked food.

I had to come up with some coping techniques to enable my students to overcome their cravings for cooked food.

Therefore I decided to create a program called "12 Steps to Raw Foods." Of course, cooked food is different from drugs or alcohol. For example, eating a slice of pizza or cake doesn't immediately and radically change one's behavior but if consumed day after day, cooked food may slowly ruin a person's health. Furthermore, consuming cooked food is not yet commonly recognized as a dependency; on the contrary, it is widely accepted and appreciated in society. That is why some of the steps in my program are different than in AA. I interviewed lots of members of various 12-Step programs, especially people from Overeaters Anonymous. These conversations helped me to create many coping techniques that I have since successfully applied in my workshops.

My first 12 Steps to Raw Foods weekend workshop was held in Portland, Oregon, in December of 1999. One month after this workshop I phoned all the participants. I was thrilled to find out that in spite of the holiday season, all forty-three people were still eating primarily raw food.

Since then I have conducted 192 weekend workshops called "12 Steps to Raw Foods" in many states and countries. These workshops became so popular that often I had more than a hundred people in the audience, sometimes two hundred. This program has proven to be considerably more effective than my initial lectures about the benefits of raw food. I felt delighted when, returning to the same town a year later, I found my students still staying 100% raw—only now they looked as if they were their own younger brothers or sisters.

12 Steps to Raw Foods workshops became profoundly impor-

tant not only for my students but also for me. These gatherings have never been merely educational events, but rather are powerful healing and learning episodes. As you may imagine, during these weekends both participants and I shared our sincere thoughts on many sensitive issues related to food. I learned a lot from these revelations. Usually, as a result of our deep communication, we all began to feel like one big family, and we even called each other "in-raws." I am so glad that I found the time to rewrite this book and to add some of the most valuable ideas that I acquired during the years of my teaching this program.

Chapter 13

HOW IMPORTANT IS IT
TO BE 100% RAW?

"To eat is a necessity, but to eat intelligently is an art."

—La Rochefoucauld

Eating a 100% raw-food diet is optimal for human health and there-fore, it is important. However, eating a 100% raw diet is not always possible. Being raised in Russia and having visited many countries, I can testify that the opportunity to eat a 100% raw vegan diet is *a luxury.* I feel fortunate to be able to eat this way. For example, I have translated my books into Russian but cannot publish them in Rus-sia because many fruits, vegetables, and especially greens are unavailable there even in the summer. I find it strange that kale originated in Russia but now it is unknown to Russian people. In the Russian version of my book I call it "wild cabbage," which can be misleading but I couldn't find a better name for it.

I also observed people unable to consume an all-raw diet due to countless other challenging situations, both in poor and wealthy countries. The following are the toughest circumstances for raw-fooders that I have encountered:

- being dependent or handicapped;
- being responsible for preparing cooked meals for other family members;

- having to eat meals prepared by other persons;
- working in a restaurant or other food-related business;
- having a severely limited availability of produce;
- dining with co-workers during business conferences;
- traveling with a group that has a pre-arranged, mostly cooked diet;
- staying in a hospital, nursing home, at war, or in prison.

Pressed with their individual limitations, people often ask my opinion on how important striving for a 100% raw regimen really is. I have two slightly different recommendations for two main kinds of eaters—compulsive eaters and normal eaters. I recommend that people try to fit themselves into one of these two types according to the following description:

- *A compulsive eater* is a person who eats more than he or she needs or wants to, not in response to signs from their stomach inciting hunger, but rather for other reasons.
- *A normal eater* is a person who eats when he or she is hungry and stops when full.[1]

If you think that you fall in between these two categories, place yourself in the group you feel closest to.

I believe that only "normal eaters" can manage to stay on a raw diet combined with small portions of cooked foods without sliding into a predominantly cooked-food diet. I would like to clarify that I don't recommend that; I only share my observation that "normal eaters" would get minimal harm from eating some cooked food because they are capable of controlling their food intake.

For compulsive eaters I strongly recommend a 100% raw-food diet simply because it would be considerably easier for them to maintain. I have observed scores of compulsive eaters attempting to stay on the combination of 80% raw and 20% cooked food. I have witnessed these poor people yo-yoing all the time from 80% raw to 80% cooked, never settling on any particular plan, always feeling guilty and worrying about their health. At the same time I have observed countless instances when, after adopting an all-raw diet, compulsive eaters were able to successfully maintain healthy eating patterns, avoid overeating, and keep breaks between meals instead of continuously grazing and snacking. Most raw foods do not possess exceedingly stimulating taste, in contrast to many cooked dishes. I have encountered some people in my life who were able to consume several large portions of pizza in one meal, but I never met anybody who could eat several large salads. Even in cases when overeating of raw products occurs, it is considerably less harmful than overeating cooked foods. Being a compulsive eater myself, I used to envy normal eaters and often felt helpless over my cravings. Staying on a 100% raw-food diet has greatly improved my eating pattern and totally transformed my entire life.

Often people ask me how 1% of cooked food in one's diet can be so harmful. I believe that when we allow 1% we leave the door open to indulge when we desire. According to AA, we tend to overeat at the times when we feel hungry, angry, lonely, tired, or depressed. Giving up the last 1% of cooked food in the diet is closing the door on cooked food altogether. When we close the door on cooked food, we close the door on temptation.

On 99% raw food, we stay vulnerable to temptation and allow ourselves what we want, when we want it. I have met many people who spent a great deal of effort to achieve the 99% raw-food level only to return to completely cooked food months later. This tiny 1% may continue to lead us back to cooked food. I consider that going "cold turkey" is much easier. Yes, one might have to suffer through the first couple of months because every temptation will create suffering. But after two months, life becomes easier.

From discussions with lots of raw-fooders I have concluded that not all cooked dishes are equally strong in triggering unnatural appetite. One should definitely stay away from all stimulating and mouth-watering cooked dishes, as well as favorite snacks. Regardless of the amount ingested, such foods could induce a powerful urge to eat more. I have watched some persons coming off a raw-food diet as a result of just one tiny bite of a cooked delicacy, after successfully staying raw for many months or even years.

At the same time, I don't want anyone to become paranoid about occasionally ingesting insignificant amounts of cooked products, especially if they are not associated with any "nostalgic" memories. For example, a few drops of pasteurized vanilla extract in one's dessert, a sheet of toasted nori, a spoonful of miso, or a pinch of nutritional yeast are not likely to stimulate one's appetite for cooked food; the body can easily handle such small occasional cooked ingredients. It is similar to a situation when an alcoholic who has quit drinking can still safely consume fried fish in a wine sauce or a slice of cake with butterscotch-flavored cream.

I believe that adopting a 100% raw-food diet is a matter of everyone's personal preference. I have several close friends and relatives for whom I know adopting a raw-food diet would be next to impossible. They would have to compromise too many of their daily values. From time to time I have presented them with nice vegan books and even steamers to encourage lighter cooking. I have noticed that they use these books and steamers and do benefit from better eating. At the same time, my friends know that if they ever wanted to make further changes in their lifestyle, I would be there to help them.

I used to think that humans could form their eating patterns throughout their entire lifetime. In my research I came upon studies about childhood imprinting. I was amazed to learn that "Flavors in mother's milk begin to shape a baby's later food preferences."[2] However, the most powerful imprint about *food preferences for life* that humans receive comes at the specific time of being weaned off mother's milk. This time is called the "sensitive period" or "critical period"[3] and lasts for two to three months during which a profoundly strong imprint is formed in every child's mind based on what the child is eating, along with watching the dining processes of other people around them, especially their mother. This imprint is practically irreversible: "A critical period . . . is very short in duration, and the effects of specific events during this period are . . . *lifelong*, and relatively *immune to erasure* by subsequent events."[4]

That is how food preferences are shaped to make us vegetarians, meat-and-potato persons, or any other kind of eater. We can become normal or compulsive eaters based on the variety of food we are exposed to during our sensitive periods. I find it fascinating that a short period of sixty to ninety days shapes eating behaviors for one's entire life. The imprint mechanism is a truly sensible way of protecting us from extinction, by making sure that the child inherits the most vital knowledge—*what to eat*—from the most caring person in the world—mother. How unfortunate it is that modern humans have stepped away from natural ways of living. By doing so, we have perverted nature's most brilliant law and have turned the advantages of lifelong healthy eating into a frustrating spell of everlasting compulsive over-consumption.

Rooted in infancy, destructive eating patterns severely undermine many people's quality of life. According to statistics, there are already 58 million Americans who are overweight[5] and these numbers are constantly growing. The scientific studies about imprinting clearly point out that it is almost impossible to overturn already existing obesity. We can see many instances where compulsive eaters desperately try to change their eating patterns. Some of them turn to such drastic solutions as undergoing gastric bypass surgery, an extreme measure that limits how much food a person can digest by stapling shut most of the stomach and cutting off ten inches of small intestine. However, nature proves to be stronger than human will power. Even after having their stomach stapled, many patients slide from the strict diet recommended by their doctors, start overeating, and regain all their weight back within five years.[6] In other words, the imprint from childhood keeps fighting for its legacy till the end. Meanwhile, a great number of people have been able to recover from obesity using a raw-food regimen and other natural ways of healing. For example, my friend Angela Stokes lost 160 pounds. She recuperated from *morbid obesity* by adopting a raw-food diet with an emphasis on greens.[7]

I think that generally, obesity is much easier to prevent than to reverse. When the water is running from the faucet onto the floor, shall we keep collecting the water with a sponge from the floorboards or close the spigot? Instead of putting all our efforts into reversing already existing obesity, let us focus on helping our children develop imprints of healthy eating. Let us pay attention to the quality and quantity of food we serve our babies, particularly during their "sensitive periods." And for the sake of shaping healthy eating patterns in our children, let us be ever mindful of the food they observe in our hands.

Chapter 14

THE ADDICTIVENESS OF COMMON FOODS

"Forget love—I'd rather fall in chocolate!"

—**Attributed to Sandra J. Dykes**

I consider a cooked-food dependency to be the cruelest of all addictions because it stems from the most desirable and even sacred foods of all humans. Bread, milk, meat, sugar, and salt are probably the most addictive of all common foods. Ironically, that is why these foods have been used for millennia and have become an essential part of human life and culture. Throughout history, whenever humans discovered an addictive substance, they never voluntarily stopped using it; furthermore, its consumption progressively continued spreading among more people. That is why all addictive matter, be it tobacco, cannabis, chocolate, or other, once discovered by one person in one country, eventually makes its way to the rest of the world. As a result, today we know of so many addictive substances that altogether they kill thousands of people and present immense social problems. We have accumulated so many foods with addictive properties that our eating choices are largely ruled by the amount of pleasure we derive from food as opposed to nutrition.

With the rapid development of new technologies, scientists have become aware of progressively more new particles in different products, including a number of addictive substances in some common foods such as sugar. Sweets taste good because eating them literally makes us feel good—sweets induce pleasurable sensations in the body. "Research indicates that sweet receptors in the mouth are coupled to brain areas that release endogenous opiates—those natural morphine-like chemicals that induce a sense of pleasure and well-being. The taste of sweet in itself is enough to activate pleasure centers in the brain."[1]

That is why most people like to consume foods that contain sugar, such as chocolate, candy, ice cream, cola, cake, and others. White sugar (or sucrose) is an unnatural molecule completely devoid of any nutritional value. At the same time, white sugar has concentrated energy and is often referred to as a source of "empty calories." Over time, ingestion of large amounts of refined sugar can lead to a "nutrient debt" wherein a person has sufficient energy to fuel the body but lacks other essential nutrients. This can result in undernourishment even in overweight persons.

In addition to eating white sugar, most people consume sucrose from cooked starchy vegetables. "In the process of cooking sweet potatoes ... nearly all of the starch present becomes converted into sugar. Thus our concept of the sweet potato as a starchy food should be revised, since when consumed by man it really is sugary rather than starchy."[2] Starchy vegetables such as potatoes, squash, carrots, broccoli, and others in a cooked form add even more sugar to our diet.

White bread, cereal, pasta, and other foods made from white flour also contain a lot of sucrose.[3] Bearing in mind that these three sources of sugar constitute the most popular fragment of the typical human diet, our consumption of sucrose is extraordinarily high, especially considering that human consumption of table sugar alone increased 4.2 times in the last hundred years.[4]

The human body tries to cope with such an enormous consumption of sugar by increasing its insulin production just after eating begins.[5] The continuous overeating of sugar inevitably leads to the condition known as hypoglycemia, when we constantly have increased levels of insulin present in our bloodstream keeping our body ready for sugar consumption at any time. Having additional insulin pumped into the blood causes abnormally low levels of blood sugar. Hypoglycemia is dangerous for the brain, which constantly needs an adequate supply of glucose. People who have hypoglycemia continuously feel the urge to eat sweets in order to level the blood sugar. Attempts to stop eating after consuming a relatively small amount usually fail due to the voracious appetite caused by this insulin-produced hypoglycemic state, thus making a binge almost inevitable. As you can see, consuming sugar in the form of sucrose inevitably leads to a dependency on sugar.

However, the body cannot function without any sugar at all. Simple sugars from fruit and honey are very easily digested and provide energy along with valuable nutrients. Ingestion of these natural sugars does not trigger the hyperglycemic response in the body.

Recently my daughter Valya and I conducted some interesting research. We decided to investigate what foods people crave in response to stress. We interviewed sixty people with specially made questionnaires. The majority (52 out of 60) of the participants reported that they crave sweets in stressful situations. However, I was more interested in the additional, unexpected information we received from our experiment. We discovered that there is a strong correlation between how people were brought up and their methods of coping with stress:

- The participants in our research who were reared on a mainstream diet admitted strong cravings for cakes, pies, cookies, candy, and other potentially hazardous sugary foods.
- People who were brought up on a vegetarian diet craved raisins, dates, and other dried fruits along with some light vegetarian desserts such as vegan whole grain muffins and licorice sticks.
- A small number of our participants grew up on a raw-food diet. I was thrilled to hear that in moments of distress, these people craved sweet fruits, such as grapes, figs, and bananas.

This investigation reminded me of the great role that childhood education plays in the development of our lifelong food preferences. My own sweetest childhood memories are always blended with pictures of eating with my family. When we look at certain food, the desire to eat it stems from our recollections of previous experiences with this food. Enjoyable memories may reinforce undesirable cravings with the longing to re-live pleasant moments once more. For example, at times when I see advertisements for pancakes, I remember my childhood and how pleasant it was to wake up on Sunday mornings to the smell of mamma's freshly made pancakes covered with melting butter. I cherish these memories, but every time they pass through my mind I experience momentary pain. I briefly feel the conflict between the subconscious urge to revive the sweet moments from the past and the notion that I won't have pancakes again because I have been eating solely raw food for many years now. It amazes me how many strong emotions can be triggered by the mere thought of food. I asked my daughter if any of her happiest childhood memories were tied to food. With a smile, she began recalling how we picked delicious grapes together in Michigan, and how the California persimmons were so yummy that even our basset hound Dashka ate so many that it was difficult for her to move, and the taste of our first durian fruit, and so on. Clearly, even though humans are programmed to crave sweets in response to stress, the sweets don't have to be made with white sugar. Fresh fruits are perfect fuel, packed with nutrients, and they don't have any negative consequences.

When I began collecting scientific data on bread I experienced a big shock and even felt pain from discovering how addictive bread really is. I lived most of my life in Russia, where bread is considered a sacred food. One can never find a piece of bread lying on the ground or on the street in Russia, because it would be considered disrespectful to all those who suffered from the shortage of bread, as in Leningrad's Blockade.* Traditionally, a sufficient supply of bread is one of the most important promises that the Russian government makes to its people. Throughout history, various breads have been a staple food for the majority of people. In the United States, November is designated National Bread Month, in recognition of the importance of this product. "More than 75 million Americans enjoy a piece of toast every day.... In fact, Americans like their toast so much that nearly 10% of adults surveyed indicated that they would rather eat toast in the morning than have sex. More than

---

*On September 8, 1941, a little over two months into the invasion of the Soviet Union, German troops surrounded Leningrad. Unable to take the city by direct assault, they set about starving it into submission. Before the siege was ended on January 27, 1944, as many as a million civilians had died from shelling, cold, and/or hunger. The Fascist blockade of Leningrad lasted nine hundred days but the city did not surrender.

half (52%) of respondents would choose toast over candy in the morning, and nearly 40% over chocolate."[6]

Have you ever wondered why bread is so popular? It may be hard to believe, but scientific research demonstrates beyond any doubt that even raw wheat contains addictive substances:

- "A novel opioid peptide was isolated from . . . wheat gluten. This peptide was named gluten exorphin C."[7]
- ". . . peptides derived from wheat gluten proteins exhibit opioid-like activity in *in vitro* tests."[8]
- "Gluten exorphins from wheat *normally* reach opiate receptors in the central nervous system and trigger their function."[9]

Scientists have measured the amount of opiates in wheat: "0.5 mg of the most active peptides were equivalent to 1 nM (nanomole) of morphine."[10] While 1 nM is only a trace amount of morphine, its quantity is still significant to the central nervous system. For example, 1 nM of morphine can be compared to the amount of opiates in our hormones such as endorphins that are synthesized by our body to combat pain or to create a feeling of pleasure and well-being. Let us also keep in mind that this amount of opiates was extracted from a very small amount of wheat.

In addition to being dependency-forming, opioid peptides from wheat also notably influence our hormonal functions: ". . . it has long been known that opioid peptides cause marked changes of pituitary hormone secretion in both animals and humans, via classical opioid receptors."[11]

I now understand why bread has been such a popular survival food for people. Due to its high sugar content, even a small piece of bread can supply one with enough energy for many hours of work. At the same time, bread has a profound calming effect through its opium-like sedating action, thus bringing satisfaction to its consumers. In addition, opioid peptides penetrate the walls of the intestines and slow down the digestion, which results in our feeling of fullness. That is why people who are accustomed to the regular eating of bread have a hard time reaching satiety without it.

However, bread, especially its white varieties, is not a nutritious food. That is why a majority of breads on the market are enriched with synthetic vitamins and minerals. Truly nutritious products don't have to be enriched. For example, I have never encountered an enriched mango or stalk of celery. Wheat contains no vitamin C, no vitamin B_{12}, no vitamin A, and no beta-carotene.[12] In countries where cereal grains comprise the bulk of the dietary intake, vitamin, mineral, and nutritional deficiencies are commonplace. Two of the major B-vitamin deficiency diseases (pellagra and beriberi) are almost exclusively associated with the excessive consumption of cereal grains.[13] In addition, I question the biological availability of most of the nutrients contained within raw grains after milling, processing, and baking.

Instead of cooking wheat and other grains, we should be sprouting them. Sprouts are living foods "enriched" by sunshine. Sprouted seeds are lower in fat than they were before germination, but have a much higher vitamin and mineral content. Most of my readers probably remember when the rumors of Y2K appeared in the late 1990s. While other people were stuffing their pantries with preserves of all kinds, my family bought only one product—a bag of organic wheat. I calculated that my family of four could have survived for approximately one year on this 50-pound bag if we consumed it in the form of sprouts.

Meat, poultry, and fish are another category of food that contains opioid peptides.[14] Some time ago, when I ate animal foods on a regular basis, I remember grilled fish and barbequed meat being my favorites. When I looked through some of the latest scientific studies on meat, I was absolutely stunned by the research conducted by Professor Matsumoto of Kanazawa University of Japan.[15] In addition to opioid peptides, AGEs, and other toxins, grilled meat contains two other toxic substances:

- 2-amino-9H-pyrido[2,3-b]indole;
- 2-amino-3-methyl-9H-pyrido[2,3-b]indole.

These toxic particles (abbreviated "AC" and "MeAC") are normally present in cigarette smoke. Professor Matsumoto determined that grilled meat has much higher concentrations of these extremely addictive substances than cigarettes. According to this research, 1g of grilled beef contains 650.8 ng of AC and 63.5 ng of MeAC, which is the equivalent of approximately 8 cigarettes. The smoke condensate of one blended cigarette contained 79.7 ng of AC and 6.2 ng of MeAC. This means that the amount of addictive toxins in one rather small 100-gram serving of barbequed meat is equal to *800 cigarettes!* It is no wonder grilled meat has been the most desired human delicacy since the beginning of cooking.

For the same reason, people tend to prefer roasted nuts over raw nuts, fried veggies over a salad, and toast over bread. We roast our cacao beans to make chocolate, and our coffee is also made of roasted beans. Some people enjoy the burning flavor of their espresso; others prefer latte, which essentially is an espresso with steamed milk added.

Milk is another product that is extremely addictive. All milk from different mammals, including human milk, naturally contains opioid peptides: "Human and bovine caseins in most species have been shown to contain, in their primary structure, peptides with opioid activity... present in the milk of all species studied so far, and is the major component of human casein micelles. It accounts for 30% of the total protein, and 70% of the casein content."[16]

The presence of addictive components in milk naturally helps build a stronger physiological connection between a mother and a baby. Such a bond is vital for the survival of a little one because it ensures that the child or the newborn nursing animal will always want to consume the most nourishing food (milk), to sleep more, and to closely follow its mother during the most vulnerable period of its life. As soon as the baby can serve itself and doesn't need to be constantly cared for by its mother, it gets weaned off mother's milk. After being weaned from milk, most existing mammals never again consume milk from their own mother or from other animals. The human is the only specie in the world that continues consuming the milk of different animals, along with other milk products, throughout life.

Due to the presence of opiates in milk, people who continue to consume milk and dairy products develop a dependency on them, especially on the most concentrated forms of dairy products, such as cheese. Most varieties of cheese also contain another addictive ingredient, salt. I continuously hear from people that cheese is one of the hardest foods to give up.

I appreciate that milk has been a survival food for millions of people throughout centuries and that without milk many would have died. I can still name a village or two in the Russian forests where there are no roads and no stores. In such conditions people depend on a cow for staying alive through the long winters. Yet that doesn't make milk the preferred nutritional choice for those who have access to more nutritious foods.

Most people add salt to every meal. While sodium *is* necessary for the proper transmission of impulses in every nerve in our body, and for muscle contraction, deficiency of sodium is difficult to achieve. Sodium salts are plentiful in the soil, and all plants grown in such soil are sufficient in sodium. No supplementation is necessary.

We should not worry about a deficiency of sodium, but rather become concerned about its excess. While the daily requirement for sodium is 50 mg, the average adult consumes 5,000 mg, a hundred times more than is needed.[17] Love of salt is an addiction similar to addictions to alcohol, tobacco, sugar, and caffeine. I found from my own experience that quitting the consumption of salt is easier than limiting it. Please note that most store-bought foods already have salt added. Being unnatural, sodium chloride impairs the salt-sensitive taste buds on our tongue to such an extent that we cannot sense most of the natural flavors of food. When one decides to quit eating salt, it usually takes only two to three days of eating bland-tasting meals before plain food seems incredibly flavorful. That is why I love eating without salt. For the same reason I believe that taking salt out of one's diet makes staying on a raw diet a lot easier.

Bread, sugar, meat, milk, and salt have been staples in the human diet for centuries, and we have become used to them. I recognize the fact that these products have played a big role in history. These foods, especially cereal grains, have enabled the survival of humans on this planet and have ultimately become responsible for the vast technological and industrial culture in which we live today. However, abundant scientific studies worldwide show us that there are better nutritional options available for humans.

In addition, there are millions of people in our world who are fortunate to have the availability of almost any food they like. I cannot find any reason for those people to continue consuming survival food. Nobody needs to wear a raincoat on a sunny day.

Chapter 15

LOOKING FOR COMFORT IN COOKED FOODS

"All happiness depends on a leisurely breakfast."

—John Gunther

"There are four basic food groups: milk chocolate, dark chocolate, white chocolate, and chocolate truffles."

—Unknown

Addictive substances in cooked foods can trigger a physical dependency on these foods. However, physical dependency is only "the tip of the iceberg." The reliance on addictive foods is often rooted in people's unaddressed needs on psychological and spiritual levels.

A psychological or mental dependency on cooked foods stems from having too much stress in combination with the habit of relaxing through eating.

We live in a stressful world. We experience stress everywhere—at school, at work, at home, in traffic, and even when we celebrate. Unfortunately, our parents and educators did not teach most of us how to handle stress properly. Instead, they taught us to eat when we experience stress:

- "Are you crying, baby? Here is a lollipop for you."
- "Honey, don't be sad, let's have some ice cream."

- "Life is so bitter, let us sweeten it with some chocolate."
- "You are going through a rough time, you deserve a treat."
- "You need to relax and eat something warm."

A connection between stress and eating is deeply ingrained in our psyches. In emotional situations, our digestive system automatically creates digestive juices, and we experience a strong need to eat something. We have even created many so-called "comfort foods." Apparently, our lives have become so stressful that we are more desperate for comfort than for nutrition.

At a local supermarket I looked through the thick food catalog and concluded that approximately 90% of all the products in the store belong to the category of comforting foods, while only about 10% are truly nutritious foods.

"Food" and "nutrition" are no longer synonyms. Consciously or subconsciously, most of us don't eat for the sake of nutrition. For example, when admiring the fancy dishes on display at the deli department, are we saying to ourselves, "Oh, the potassium in that cheesecake is calling my name!" If we ate solely for nutritional purposes, we would never put into our mouths such harmful things as candy, chips, popcorn, or pizza. None of us is suffering from a pizza deficiency, but it is one of the most popular foods. Popcorn is not nutritious, but it gives us comfort when the movie is boring. Chips are overloaded with salt and saturated fat, but they help us stay awake while driving. It is the pleasure and comfort that we anticipate from the food and rarely its nutrition.

According to *WordNet* (an online dictionary), "comforting" means "providing freedom from worry."[1] While exploring which foods most people consider to fit the category of "providing freedom from worry," I found a list of the ten most popular comforting foods in the United Kingdom, published by BBC.[2] As you can see, these are not very nutritious choices:

1. chocolate
2. cup of tea
3. toast
4. ice cream
5. sausage, egg, chips, and beans
6. sausage and mash
7. soup
8. fruit crumble pie
9. sponge pudding
10. rice pudding

Eating in order to nourish our emotional needs, to calm stress, or to have a break from empty feelings has become almost normal. Many restaurants, retreats, and cookbooks promote their foods as "comforting." Yet the main purpose of eating *is* nutrition. Only the consumption of nutrient-rich food ensures optimal health. There can be no compromise. If we live in a stressful world, let us create techniques for handling stress that are different from eating comforting food.

I consider walking to be an effective natural way of handling stress. If you don't like walking, you may practice other forms of exercise. I prefer walking because it is the most natural movement for all humans and is good both for the mind and the body. Walking relieves stress because it provides a way for the body to release tension and built-up frustration by raising the output of endorphins—one of the "feel good" chemicals in the brain. I notice that dog owners who walk their dogs daily are generally well-balanced people. When my friend lost his dog he kept walking every day out of habit as if he still had a dog. Therefore, walk your dog every day, even if you don't have one.

All healthy children naturally want to walk or run when they are stressed. Parents often feel nervous when children run around or jump in our restricted environment. So we tie our children to strollers, car seats, and shopping carts for safety. And to control their stress we offer them treats.

When I was a child, my family was so poor that I owned only one dress, which was also my school dress. Nevertheless, my parents made sure we had enough bread, milk, eggs, cheese, meat, and even a chocolate cake once in a while. Eating was important and it certainly was pleasant. I remember always chewing something when I was reading a book or watching TV. This habit has stayed with me until now. Whenever I read or watch a movie my hands search for something to grab and my mouth waters. Sometimes I am able to suppress this craving, but often I eat an apple or chunks of vegetables.

I have been fortunate in my life to meet such rare people as my friends Vanessa and Jonathan, who don't seem to have attachments to any foods. They told me that their mothers didn't make food the center of their life. Jonathan's mother would never call him to eat if he was busy playing. She figured that playing was more important for life than eating. As a result, his life is not centered on food. He tells me he can go for hours without thinking of food. Vanessa has little memory of how chocolate, salmon, white bread, or Coca Cola taste. She was raised on a vegan diet. Once in a while, at her friends' houses she was offered other food, but after trying it she preferred to wait till she got home because her mother's healthy food tasted a lot better to her. Vanessa was amazed at how the opposite was true for her friends.

Most people cannot imagine living without delicious cooked meals. For this reason the beginning raw-fooders often look for dishes that closely remind them of the tastes of their favorite cooked dishes. Many raw recipes have names such as "un-burrito," "mock chocolate," "like-tuna sandwich," and so on. However, raw foods don't have addictive substances in them and thus cannot "provide freedom from worry." That is why carob candy cannot completely satisfy our craving for chocolate. Even when we are able to achieve a wonderful taste with raw food, we still don't get the result we were longing for, in terms of our emotional needs. There is only one circumstance in which raw food may give an enormous pleasure and satisfaction, and that is when we are truly hungry. Hence, for those who are used to grazing all day long, raw meals might not provide the sought-after comfort. That is why it is essential for everyone to find ways other than food to cope with stress, particularly when adopting a raw way of eating. I know too many people who successfully stayed on a raw-food regimen for a long time and then suddenly slipped off their diet, unable to handle pressure. Some of my friends admitted that sliding back to cooked food aggravated their stress even further because it caused a drop in their energy levels and made them overall less vibrant. On the other hand, applying stress-handling techniques might have helped them to live through their emotional catastrophes without sliding off their raw-food plans.

Chapter 16

FEEDING INNER HUNGER

"Happiness is the ability to feel endless beauty in every moment."

—Igor Boutenko

We have already discussed the dependency on cooked foods on physical and psychological levels. Now I would like to talk about the level of addiction that is hardest to overcome—the spiritual level. How can we battle our deep spiritual emptiness?

Many of my students have told me that they often eat in an attempt to numb the unbearable empty feelings they experience. They also comment that trying to fill that emptiness and depression with food only deepens the hole further. I understand that the feelings of spiritual emptiness and depression have a lot in common. Below are some statistics on depression.

- Depressive disorders affect approximately 18.8 million American adults or about 9.5% of the U.S. population age 18 and older in a given year.[1]
- Everyone will at some time in their life be affected by depression—their own or someone else's—according to Australian government statistics. (Depression statistics in Australia are comparable to those of the U.S. and U.K.)[2]

- The rate of increase of depression among children is an astounding 23% per year.[3]
- 30% of women are depressed. Men's figures were previously thought to be half that of women, but new estimates are higher.[4]
- 15% of depressed people will commit suicide.[5]
- In 2002, 31,655 (approximately 11 per 100,000) people died by suicide in the U.S.[6]
- Antidepressants work only as well (or less) than placebos.[7, 8]

As you can see, depression is one of the greatest problems of our time, claiming the lives of millions. Many professional psychiatrists consider that the optimal treatment for depression is fostering spiritual beliefs, developing a sense of purpose, and sharing those experiences with others.[9, 10]

Most of the existing 12-Step programs, such as AA, NA, and OA, are spiritual in their nature, and "if these programs are practiced as a way of life, can expel the obsession to use the substance of abuse and enable the sufferer to become happy and useful and whole."[11] At least eleven thousand addiction treatment programs in the United States introduce their clients to some form of spirituality.[12]

The 12-Step programs lead an alcoholic or an addict to admit the problem, turn to a higher power (or "God, as we understand him"), make amends, pray, and meditate. Other programs offer alternative spiritualities, such as Yoga, Islam, or Native American religions. There are also programs that encourage members to follow their own religion.

The word "spiritual" originates from "spirit," which is equivalent to the Latin word *spiritus*, a breath. "Spirit" has the same meaning in Russian: "douh"—a "breath." Similarly, life enters the human body with a first breath and leaves the body with a last breath. According to *Webster's Dictionary*, the word "spiritual" means "the quality or state of being."[13] Therefore, spirituality is not just a belief because beliefs alone do not create a spiritual *state of being*, although beliefs may (and often do) lead to values through personal verification.

I trust that all humans are spiritual beings. When people don't feel spirituality, they often develop feelings of the pointlessness of their mere existence. As a result, they develop low drive for life and become depressed. Certainly, a pill cannot reassure a person in his or her values of life. That is why developing spirituality, not pharmacology or will power, underlies a successful recovery from addiction.

Unfortunately, there are endless controversies surrounding faith-based treatment, from the conflict between science and spirituality, to the skepticism about the "New Age" brand of spirituality (which many of these programs encourage), to constitutional issues over court-mandated participation in allegedly religious treatment programs.[14] If our goal is helping people end their suffering, we should be focusing on the results rather than the validity of one or the other belief. If we could expand on the idea of spirituality beyond the doctrinal and ritualistic form to a wider range of thought, it would enable many more people to embrace spirituality.

Even finding a spiritual foundation cannot guarantee that faith-based comfort will not fade away. I know firsthand that the feeling of spiritual emptiness can often come to those who already recognize the spirituality of the universe as a reality. I have heard from many friends that the hardest part for them was to remain connected to their spiritual beliefs, especially in situations where people observed some kind of injustice. I believe that all people in the world were initially kind, considerate persons. In his book *The Brighter Side of Human Nature,* Alfie Kohn draws from hundreds of compelling studies in psychology, sociology, economics, and biology to demonstrate convincingly that we are more caring than we give ourselves credit for, and that our generosity cannot be reduced to mere self-interest. Kohn, for example, points out how early in life we begin responding to others' distress, and that humans are the only animals who can choose to look at the world from another being's perspective.[15] I witness compassion of human nature whenever I visit the movie theater. Watching the depth of empathy that the audience develops towards the strangers on the screen reveals how sensitive we all are to the pain and joy of others. If the main character suffers, one may glance back at the audience to find a sea of sad and tearful faces, while during a happy film, the viewers often smile and leave in high spirits.

There is a lot of distraction happening in today's world. When confronted by an avalanche of negative reports, we might begin to think that the world is unfair. Witnessing unfairness creates an assault on our emotions and our intellects. Disconnecting from our ideals, we may feel like orphans, starved for the nourishment of the soul. We then try eating some delicious, comforting food but it doesn't help, as we continue to be spiritually undernourished.

At the same time, there is a higher justice, higher power, higher love, and higher beauty in the universe. It is reflected in every human being and in every piece of nature. Noticing these reflections of an invisible yet powerful spiritual realm always helps me restore my own strength, balance, and happiness. The message from the spiritual universe may arrive merely through someone's warm glance, someone's gentle touch, the kiss of a child, or the stunning cuteness of a puppy. Similar experiences remind us that material force is not the only power in the world. I cannot describe in words what exactly takes place when those moments happen. I only know that since I have learned to be more attentive to these *little* episodes in my life, I don't fall into emotional lows and powerlessness anymore. Instead, I have gained my personal balance in which I feel connected to the core of my being and to the wisdom and power of spirituality. I know that all people have different names for these precious powers. I consider that a name is not as important as the true notion that all humans are spiritual beings.

Part 3

HOW TO END YOUR DEPENDENCY ON COOKED FOOD

BECOMING AWARE OF THE PROBLEM

"And ye shall know the truth, and the truth shall set you free."

—John 8:32

The first and probably the most difficult step is to closely observe oneself, to explore if one has a dependency on cooked food, to evaluate the level of this dependency, and to admit that there is a problem. We cannot fix a problem without knowing what the trouble is. To diagnose correctly is very important. Imagine that your car has stopped in the middle of a bridge. You wouldn't start changing the tires or pulling the engine apart without specifying the problem first. Most likely, you would gladly pay money just for the diagnosis alone.

Similarly, when people feel the need to quit eating certain foods, and they have not yet realized they have developed a dependency on these foods, they start acting without adequate tools and are likely to fail. In order to help you clarify for yourself whether you are able to manage your eating habits, I have developed a special questionnaire.

Cooked Food Dependency Questionnaire

Please answer "Yes" or "No" to each of the following questions. If you want to answer "Sometimes," "Maybe," or "Rarely" then answer "Yes." Please be honest.

1. If you are not hungry, but someone offers you your favorite delicious food, do you accept the offer?
2. If you know that it is not good to eat before bedtime, but there is some delicious food on the table, do you eat it?
3. Do you eat more food than usual when you are stressed?
4. Do you continue eating until your stomach feels completely full?
5. Do you eat when you are bored?
6. Do you notice restaurant signs even when you are not hungry?
7. If you are made an offer for a free dinner, do you always accept the offer?
8. Do you usually overeat at all-you-can-eat restaurants?
9. Have you ever broken a promise to yourself not to eat before bedtime?
10. Would you spend the last $10 in your pocket on your favorite food?
11. Do you reward yourself with food for accomplishing achievements?
12. Do you eat extra food rather than letting it go to waste?
13. If you know that eating a certain food you really enjoy will make you feel ill later, do you still eat it?

If you answered "Yes" to three or more questions, then you may have a dependency on cooked food.

Raw-fooders also sometimes answer "Yes" to more than three questions. For several months and even years after adopting a raw-food diet, most people continue viewing food as a comforting element. Then, little by little, they begin to create other sources of comfort and pleasure in their lives, and their focus might shift away from food after a while.

In this first step we are only searching for an indication of a dependency in our eating patterns. If you notice signs of it, please observe your behavior without any judgment, feelings of guilt, or remorse. This program is not aimed at dumping your self-esteem, but rather finding the best possible ways of coping with your eating habits, and eventually building up healthy relationships with food. This is only the first step.

Here is another questionnaire for you. Please answer the following three questions. It is very important that you do so quickly and honestly. It is even better if you answer these questions with a friend.

1. Have you ever overeaten in your life? Yes or No?
2. Did you like how you felt afterwards? Yes or No?
3. Can you promise me here and now that you will never do it again? Yes or No?

To tell you the truth, I have yet to meet the lucky person who has never overeaten in his/her life. If you are not that fortunate being, then please try to recollect in detail your bodily experiences after a big meal. Perhaps you didn't like how you felt after overeating. You probably felt as if you had a brick in your stomach, had nightmares later that night, and looked puffy the next morning. Maybe you even swore to never overeat again. But when I ask if you would do it again, you will most likely nod, "Yes!"

Often we act as if food has become our main pleasure. To celebrate our birthdays, anniversaries, or other occasions, we organize fancy and abundant feasts. When we attend a birthday party, we expect to be nicely fed. How would you feel about a party where no food was offered?

"Food" has become synonymous with "celebration" and "enjoyment." For holiday dinners we plan delicious meals, spend extra money, and prepare the most mouth-watering items to eat. We even have an arsenal of special festive dishes such as tortes, chocolate truffles, ice cream, and candy, along with an extended assortment of appetizers. Often we look forward to eating as if it were the most essential part of the entire celebration.

We try not to think of how we are going to feel the next morning. Naturally after a big party we feel tired, sleepy, and even sick. In many cases we attempt to fix our poor condition with coffee or medicine. However, all this suffering doesn't stop us from planning our next holiday meal. Such an irrational performance clearly demonstrates many people's inability to manage their eating behavior, or in other words, a dependency.

To better understand any possible challenges you may have encountered in the past in your efforts to maintain a healthy diet, let us bring to light some of your previous experiences with food. Please answer the following questions, preferably on paper. Take your time, as you need to collect as much information as possible to properly evaluate your relationships with food.

1. Have you ever tried to quit eating any particular food (bread, chocolate, meat, popcorn, ice cream, coffee, cheese, sugar, etc.)? Yes or No?
2. Did you try to stop eating this food more than once? Yes or No?
3. If yes, can you think of why you had to make more than one attempt?

To quit eating certain foods is not as easy as it seems, even in cases of lethal danger. We all are aware of people who undergo life-threatening surgeries, have their stomachs stapled, take questionable diet pills, or smoke dangerous substances to suppress their appetites. Millions of others force themselves to throw up after they overeat, or fast for a few days on water, only to go back to binging. If there were no dependency on cooked foods, these drastic measures would be unnecessary.

Once I was helping for nine months as a volunteer at the Creative Health Institute (CHI) in Michigan. During this time 132 people who had cancer went through the program at CHI. All these people were placed on a strict raw-food diet with an emphasis on greens and sprouts (a diet developed by Dr. Ann Wigmore—see Chapter 3). Most of these guests felt better within a matter of weeks. Their tumors began to shrink, and they had more energy. Some of them even applied for new jobs and submitted applications to college. When our guests returned home, they continued on this diet for a while. But when the holidays came, they *all* slipped off. All of these people died because they couldn't stay on a raw-food diet. They left children and loved ones behind because they were not able to resist their cravings for cooked food. I knew each one of those people personally. I was teaching them to grow sprouts and drink wheatgrass juice. I talked to their families, which were supportive because they witnessed a positive change in the health of their loved ones. I especially remember Cynthia, a thirty-year-old schoolteacher who had solid support from her whole family. Her three sons pleaded, "Mom, we're going to make juice for you. Just stay on this raw-food diet and stay alive." Her husband said, "Stay raw, we will eat with you." She couldn't stay on the raw-food diet.

Her cancer came back. Cynthia sent me a "Thank You" note before she died.

These stories show that a dependency on cooked food is often stronger than fear of death. It is more powerful than the fear of disease, no matter how great the suffering and pain. Understanding how addictive cooked food can be helps conquer this dependency. The following exercise is instrumental in finding additional information about your eating patterns that are not always obvious.

On a new page in your notebook, try to remember a minimum of five instances when you were hiding from others what you were eating.

To help you with ideas, read some examples from my workshops, written by my students:

Erica: During Halloween, I tried to eat my children's candy when they were at school "so that they would have less sugar for themselves."

Matt: I'd been trying to stay raw for six months already. Then my sister visited me and brought my favorite donuts from Puck's, wrapped in cellophane. In the middle of the night when everybody was sleeping, I went to the kitchen and decided to eat one. But the cellophane made this crackling sound, and it was so loud, I was afraid everybody in the house would wake up. However, I managed to eat three of them without being noticed.

Helen: I never buy cooked food, but when I go to the store, I go for the bulk bins and sneak a candy. Sometimes I circle around the store, coming back for another piece.

Tony: My wife and I had been sticking to raw food now for three months. And then my co-worker brought pizza for lunch. The smell of it got to me and I couldn't stop thinking about it. So after work on the way home I drove through Pizza Hut and bought myself a slice. I didn't want my wife to know that I'd had pizza because I was afraid she would want some too. So on the way home I stopped and threw away the wrappers. Then I had a horrible aftertaste and it was not even as good as I had expected.

Ann: I had been raw for one month, and my husband was not supportive. He constantly made fun of me. My resolve weakened, and I started to crave muffins. I decided to eat one, but I didn't want anyone to know, so I drove to a bakery I knew on the other side of town. I bought a muffin and ate it inside, looking carefully to make sure there were no acquaintances in sight. I disposed of the wrapper but forgot about the crumbles on my dark raincoat. When I came home my husband instantly asked me, "Ann, did you have a muffin?"

I cried out, "Have you been spying on me?"

He replied, "There are crumbles on your raincoat!"

I turned red.

Rebecca: I invited Victoria to stay in our house after a workshop. So I decided to clean my pantry. I had there some boxes of cereal that were not raw, and I didn't want her to see them.

Ingrid: I have been on and off raw food for almost a year now. About once a month I begin to crave fried potato skins, home fries from the deli that come in a box. I pick them up and put them under my car seat. Then I go to pick up my son from day care. It's a long drive home, about thirty minutes, and I usually can't wait, but I don't want my son to see me eating those, or he would ask me for some and I know they are not good for him. Since he is strapped in the toddler seat right behind me, I manage to eat without him seeing, and I polish the entire box off before we get home. I feel so stupid doing this, plus my fingers get sticky and I have to clean the steering wheel. But for some reason it happens again and again.

Jessica: At my work in my office, I have chocolate candies hidden deep in my desk cabinet behind all the papers. When no one is looking I eat them.

Lucy: I have been perfectly raw for six weeks, and my family supports me. So when we went to a family reunion, they let me prepare my own food and they didn't push me to eat their food. It was very hard for me to look at my favorite dishes from childhood, vegan though not raw, but I managed not to touch them. However, in the middle of the night I went to the kitchen where there were dishes that had some leftovers, and I gobbled them. Then I went back to sleep.

Bob: I used to be a great vegetarian cook. So after I'd been on raw food for almost two months, my friends asked me if I could prepare them my best dish, cheese dumplings with mushroom cream sauce. It was my best friend's birthday, so I decided to do so. The morning of the birthday, I started cooking. While I was waiting for the dumplings to boil, I decided I needed to try the sauce to make sure it was exactly right. I tried it again and again until there was so little left, it was not enough to serve, so I decided to finish it. While my friends were eating the dumplings without the sauce, they kept saying how good it was, but how wonderful it would have been to have the sauce.

I practice this exercise in many of my workshops. After each testimony, I ask the rest of the group, "How many of you can relate to this story?" Almost everyone in the entire audience raises her or his hand. I find this exercise helpful for a more thorough observation of the variety of behavioral patterns surrounding foods. This exercise is instrumental in estimating our level of dependency on certain foods, because it helps us recognize that it was our craving for a particular food that forced us to perform such weird actions as hiding, lying, and even stealing food. It is always helpful to understand the real motives behind those actions and to become aware of the severity of our personal addiction.

I have noticed that it also brings a sense of relief and even elevates participants' self-esteem when they realize that attempts to hide one's eating patterns are rather typical for many people. Most people have tried to eat healthier and have failed at least once. As a result, they begin to subconsciously believe they are not good enough, and that they should know better. I believe that any guilt is unnecessary and destructive. Instead of wasting time feeling guilty, let us perform the necessary steps to eliminate these harmful habits.

Let us start observing our actions, and especially our thoughts. For example, pay attention to how we choose one food over another. Perhaps at the health food store we see an organic mango and it's, "Oh boy!"—$2.99 for one piece. Often we think, "How expensive!" Then we turn around to the deli and see freshly baked croissants for $2.99. We think, "Oh, what a good deal, I'm hungry." It is helpful to find out what reasoning compels us to choose a nutritionally poor croissant over a piece of nourishing fruit. Possibly we long for quick pleasure, or strive to numb an empty feeling inside, and that mango might not bring us an expected satisfaction but the croissant will. According to research done at Cornell University, when people have a dependency, they feel a strong need to consume a certain substance not to feel pleasure, or a high, but *merely to feel satisfied,* or to function normally.[1] If this is the case with choosing a croissant, then the sooner we recognize the problem, the better.

The process of becoming aware of one's dependency can be so painful that people call it "hitting rock bottom." Maybe you have heard that one has to "hit rock bottom" in order to end an addiction. Perhaps you know some persons who drank for many years, ruined their health, lost their families and jobs, their loved ones begging them to quit but they couldn't. Then suddenly they "hit rock bottom" and a miracle happened: they became sober for good. Have you ever thought of what makes that "rock bottom" such a powerful place? I used to think that finding "rock bottom" depends on the depth of despair or even closeness to death. Then I noticed that everyone hits his or her "rock bottom" at different levels of addiction. Some people get emphysema before they quit smoking; some are able to quit at a very early stage of addiction; and some lose everything and die but never quit. That means that hitting the "rock bottom" is not connected to disease and despair but to something else. What is that magic wand that returns people to the fullness of life?

The miraculous transformation happens when a person perceives the problem so clearly that he/she is not afraid to admit it to others. That is why admitting the dependency is the core of all the 12-Step programs. Often it takes a lifetime of suffering before a person arrives at the point of awareness of their real problem. Some people are afraid of admitting the truth; others don't understand why it is so important. You probably have heard some alcoholics say, "I can stop drinking any time I want. I just drink to relax." Or maybe you have heard smokers declare, "I can quit smoking but I really enjoy it and I feel fine."

Such non-willingness to acknowledge the truth is called *denial*. We all know that smoking and drinking are harmful to the body, but people in denial are rejecting those obvious facts, and this breeds their further disorientation. On the other hand, admitting the truth creates relief and eliminates confusion. By admitting our problem, we achieve clarity about what to do next and gain the power needed for further steps. There is no need to get into deep sorrow or become desperately ill in order to make a change—let us hit "rock bottom" sooner rather than later.

When we have a correct diagnosis, we can start the positive transformation. The power is in knowing oneself.

NOURISHING YOUR BODY TO ELIMINATE CRAVINGS

"He that takes medicine and neglects diet wastes the skill of the physician."

—**Chinese Proverb**

During the last two hundred years, humans have been consuming an increasingly larger percentage of highly processed, devitalized foods. As a result, many people have become chronically malnourished. That is why, regardless of our undeniable success in medicine, today's statistics on human health are frightening: "Within a decade, America will spend one of every five dollars on health care, according to government analysts. . . . The nation's total health care bill by 2015 will be more than $4 trillion."[1]

I believe that the epidemics of degenerative disease experienced today are rooted in the lack of proper nutrition that has already lasted for an extensive period of time. The numbers for degenerative disease and obesity are especially alarming in well-developed countries, where the population consumes large amounts of refined foods.

To cope with the malnourishment, the human body creates an additional urge to eat, and we begin feeling constantly hungry. Our cells are "crying" for all the nutrients we need. Sadly, we respond to this urge by eating more processed food, which promotes even further malnourishment, along with an increased dependency on processed food, greater cravings, and compulsive eating. For anyone involved in such a vicious cycle, the conversion to a raw-food diet appears to be extremely difficult because of the constant appetite. That is why I recommend nourishing your body for several weeks before switching to a raw-food diet.

I consider greens to be the top nutritious food on Earth. Blending is similar to chewing; therefore, eating blended food can make a dramatic improvement in your health. After being broken down in a high-speed blender, pieces of food become the perfect size for assimilation. Therefore, green smoothies are the best food to aid in a rapid restoration of the body's nutrient reserves. Recovering from inadequate nutrition will significantly reduce unhealthy cravings and prepare you for an easier transition to the raw-food lifestyle. In some cases natural supplements could be useful; however, I would like to caution against trying to substitute supplements for real food. The regular consumption of nutritionally rich whole foods will ease your cravings and enable your dietary transition.

I highly recommend consuming green smoothies on a regular basis, whether on a raw or cooked-food diet. I have already witnessed many cases in which people were able to greatly improve their health by adding blended greens to their daily regimen. From my observation, the best results are achieved by substituting a quart of green smoothie for your breakfast meal.

Following are testimonials from people whose cravings were decreased or even eliminated by consuming green smoothies.

"My boyfriend and I have slowly been making our way towards foods that are alive, but we have been struggling. And then we began drinking these green smoothies. Now, after my food cravings have diminished, my toenail fungus has vanished, and my acne is a past memory . . . we are happier, calmer, and loving our daily green smoothies. They made a dramatic impact on our family. I would recommend drinking green smoothies to everyone."—Natalie

"For the past twenty years I've been on a quest to eat more natural foods, and my health improved drastically. But I still suffered from junk food cravings . . . until I discovered green smoothies. Now my cravings are totally gone!"—Robin

"Following Victoria's advice, I added lots of greens to my fruit smoothies, and the first day I did so my food cravings stopped. Bang. Just vanished. It was as if my brain's 'cravings switch' was flipped to the 'Off' position. Apparently my body had been craving minerals all those years, and once I started eating greens, the cravings stopped. I'm finally trimming down!"—Robert

"My wife and I surely love the changes that are happening in our bodies! Make yourself some green smoothies, and watch your food cravings vanish. This is the secret to losing weight!"—Mark

"'The green smoothies are delicious. Yes, I like greens anyway, but I have personally witnessed non-greens lovers actually enjoying the smoothies I make. These same Standard American Diet people now regularly request large helpings of raw fruits and vegetables. What an easy way to make a difference in people's lives!"—Laura B.

Add green smoothies to your regular diet until you notice that you begin to naturally desire salads, fruits, and other raw foods. When you notice that cravings for your favorite cooked dishes become milder and more tolerable, you may consider yourself ready to transition to a raw-food diet.

You will find several delicious recipes for green smoothies at the end of this book. Please note that these recipes are provided just as basic ideas. Feel free to substitute fruits and greens to increase your variety.

ACQUIRING SKILLS AND EQUIPMENT

"Cooking is like love. It should be entered into with abandon or not at all."

—**Harriet van Horne**

If you have seriously decided to adopt a raw-food diet as your primary way of eating, acquiring raw-food preparation skills is of foremost importance. It doesn't matter if you have a raw-food restaurant on your block or if your spouse is an accomplished raw gourmet chef. After many years of observation, I came to the conclusion that every raw-fooder who depends on others for his or her daily meals is less likely to remain on a raw-food diet while drifting through different life challenges.

I have taught thousands of people to prepare delicious raw gourmet concoctions, and I know that the absolute majority of people are capable of learning the basic skills of raw cuisine fairly quickly and easily.

First, I would like to explain why such expertise is so important. People on a typical cooked-food diet consume more or less the same things every day. For example, be it a steak, or goulash, or burger, or barbeque, it is still beef, even though it appears differently. Even when substituted with chicken, pork, or fish, all meats have a similar taste, texture, and nutritional content (except for the amount of fat, which may vary depending on the quality). I bet most consumers wouldn't be able to distinguish between the taste of a beef, pork, or chicken hot dog, or even between a chicken or tofu burger if the same seasonings were used.

Foods that are typically eaten with meat, such as fried potatoes, baked potatoes, mashed potatoes, rice, pasta, or bread, consist of mostly carbohydrates and fat, and these are also very similar in their taste and nutritional value. Of course, adding raw vegetables to a meal would create a major nutritional improvement, but unfortunately that is still a rare occurrence: "When Americans dined out in 2005, the leading menu choices remained hamburgers, french fries, and pizza. The presumably healthier option of a side salad was the No. 4 choice for women, and No. 5 for men, according to the eating pattern study."[1]

In contrast, there is a wide variety of fresh produce available in this country. Each supermarket in the U.S. carries a variety of 130 fruits and 196 vegetables throughout the year.[2] Raw, uncooked vegetables, greens, fruits, nuts, and seeds all possess their own unique flavor.

To cook an unusual gourmet dish with such monotonous ingredients as meat and potatoes, one has to be an experienced and gifted chef. The epicurean tastes of a cooked diet are typically achieved through enhancing recipes with complex combinations of herbs and condiments, without which the dish would taste bland. For the convenience of consumers, who generally lack such skills, there are many premixed cooked foods sold in supermarkets. To keep the food cost down, the main condiments used in those packages are narrowed down to salt and pepper. To increase the shelf life, preservatives are added. The typical diet of citizens living in industrialized countries consists primarily of a combination of pre-cooked or partially cooked packaged foods. Meanwhile, "Fewer than 1/3 of all meals prepared at home are made from 'scratch'."[3]

In contrast, preparing a raw-food meal requires merely basic skills, and the taste of raw food is determined not by condiments but rather by the diversity of natural flavors of vegetables, greens, fruits, nuts, herbs, etc. For example, take a recipe, "I Can't Believe It's Just Cabbage," from this book.* There are only three ingredients in this recipe: cabbage, oil, and salt. Yet I have been successfully serving this dish at many gatherings, for guests with various food preferences, and even to my gourmet meat-eating relatives. Everyone loves it. I am constantly observing people being amused by the unexpectedly scrumptious taste of raw cuisine.

Tired of the rather boring taste of cooked dishes and longing for tasty, nostalgic, homey, or authentic dishes, people go out with increasing frequency: "In 2005 there were 925,000 restaurants in U.S., serving more than 70 billion meals and snacks. Having 12.5 million employees, the industry is the largest employer besides government."[4]

According to *ABC News*, "Americans are eating out at restaurants increasingly more often. Statistics show that the average household spends 40% of its food dollar eating away from home."[5]

However, food in most restaurants is far from being "nostalgic, homey, and authentic." Due to soaring prices of high-quality ingredients, the high cost of services of professional chefs, and tough competition in the restaurant business, increasingly more restau-

---

*Please see the recipe in Part 4 of this book.

rants adopt a fast-food style of preparing meals. The statistics for just three popular fast-food franchises follow:

- Total number of Subway restaurants in the U.S. in July 2006 was 20,000.[6]
- Total number of McDonald's outlets in the U.S. in 2005 was 12,658.[7]
- Total number of Wendy's restaurants in the U.S. in 2005 was 5,840.[8]

Given that I stayed for many years first on cooked and then on the raw-food diet, I have had a chance to compare the two ways of eating. I noticed that these two eating patterns required my body to perform in two different ways. I think that when I ate mostly cooked food, I almost never satisfied my bodily requirements for nutrition. Therefore, my decisions about how much food to consume in one meal were not determined by the amount of nutrients from this meal but rather by the feeling of fullness in my stomach and possibly by fulfilling my cravings that stemmed from a dependency on certain foods. Since I adopted a raw-food lifestyle, my appetite often stops while I am only in the middle of my plate and I feel completely fed and satisfied *despite* the absence of a full feeling in my belly.

There is also a big difference between motives that drive raw- or cooked-food diners to make their food choices. I discovered this diversity while conducting an experiment in one of my classes, when I interviewed about forty of my students, both cooked- and raw-food eaters. I asked everyone a simple question: "What is your favorite meal?" Most of the people on a cooked-food diet knew exactly what their most wanted dishes were, along with many details, such as which sauce had to accompany this dish or at which restaurant the meal was served. Unexpectedly, all of the respondents who ate raw food named dozens of favorite recipes, fruits, vegetables, berries, nuts, and so on. In addition, many of them mentioned that their favorite foods were constantly changing; others enjoyed particular foods only when they were in season.

I concluded that people eating mostly cooked food are driven in their desire to eat largely by the taste of food, by their possible dependency on particular foods, and on rare occasions by their bodily nutritional demands. By comparison, raw-food eaters are generally motivated by particular nutrients in certain produce. That is why their preference keeps adjusting to the changing of their bodily nutritional demands.

I hope that after reading all these facts and observations you will understand why it is vitally important for every raw-fooder to be capable of preparing her or his own meals.

I have observed that most people who implement a raw-food lifestyle pass through three main stages:

1. **The transitional stage.** During this time, which may last from a couple of months to a couple of years, people consume a lot of so-called "raw gourmet foods" that usually contain lots of nuts, oils, and condiments, and are not made according to the rules of proper food combining.* Raw gourmet dishes traditionally have names and appearances that resemble popular cooked recipes, such as "Un-burrito," "Nice Cream," or "Rawsage." You will

---

*Food combining was first described in the early twentieth century by Dr. William Howard Hay. Its principles encourage separating specific foods, eating certain ones together, and only in specified meals.

encounter a lot of these dishes in raw-food restaurants and at raw-food festivals. The food during this stage is somewhat comforting due to its heaviness and gourmet taste, and therefore such foods help to overcome the dependency on cooked foods. Many people crave a lot of flax crackers and other dehydrated foods during this stage. You don't have to learn how to prepare many different gourmet recipes unless you want to, but I highly recommend learning three or four basic recipes.

2. **The Salad Stage.** At a certain point in your raw-food life, you will begin to naturally crave simpler dishes as opposed to those heavy gourmet concoctions. From this time on, little by little, salads will become your staple for a long time, possibly for years. An endless variety of salads with some fruits and nuts or seeds will totally satisfy your needs for calories, nutrition, and pleasure.

3. **The Whole-Foods Stage.** People usually arrive at this stage after many years of living on a raw-food diet. During this phase you will naturally prefer whole foods to salads. You will develop a strong preference for the highest-quality seasonal ripe fruits and vegetables. You will most likely stop or greatly reduce your consumption of oils, sweeteners, and dehydrated foods. You will always crave exactly what your body needs for your health, and you will consume those precious foods with heavenly enjoyment. I don't know yet if there are more stages after this one.

Don't rush or pull yourself through these stages; rather, follow your bodily intuitive guidance. That will ensure your happy thriving on a raw-food diet.

Following are nine main advantages of being self-reliant in terms of preparing raw meals:

- You will always be well fed no matter where you are.
- You can individualize your diet based on your personal cravings to ensure the adequate nourishing of your body.
- You will always eat delicious food of your own choice.
- You will be able to quickly adjust your diet according to your personal transitions from one stage to another.
- Your skills in preparing a couple of perfected, scrumptious raw gourmet dishes will enable you to pleasantly surprise your guests and will attract more like-minded friends into your social life.
- You will always be appreciated at raw and vegan potlucks.
- Your dining will always be most economical.
- You won't have to depend on others to be fed.
- You can teach raw culinary arts to many others.

Start with obtaining the necessary raw kitchen appliances. The following is my family's favorite raw-food kitchen equipment.

• Vita-Mix Blender

After many years of preparing raw dishes and trying various blenders, we have concluded that the Vita-Mix is the best. It is super-powerful and reliable. This heavy-duty blender can almost liquefy wooden blocks.

• Champion Juicer

We use the versatile Champion to make juices, purées, pâtés, and ice creams. The Champion is a very practical juicer because it is easy to use and clean.

• Cuisinart

This food processor is absolutely the best because it lasts forever and has high-quality blades that don't get dull. The Cuisinart grinds hard vegetables, nuts, and seeds that give other food processors trouble.

• Excalibur Dehydrator

We like this dehydrator because it dries crackers, cookies, and veggies evenly and thoroughly. It conveniently opens in the front and has a thermostat that you can set to low temperatures. We recommend the nine-tray version even for one person because no one would want to make a new batch of crackers every day.

• Milk Bag/Sprout Bag

We use these bags to strain nut and seed milks and also for sprouting seeds and beans. You may make your own nut milk bag out of nylon fabric or buy one through our website: www.rawfamily.com.

Begin using your new tools. It's impossible to turn into a raw chef by merely watching accomplished chefs, just as it is impossible to turn into a good swimmer by observing Olympic swimmers. Pick one or two recipes, buy the ingredients, and start practicing. If your creation doesn't taste good yet, you may put it in your compost. All the earthworms from your neighborhood will gather in your garden, attracted by your cuisine.

I remember how I couldn't convince my husband to help me make garden burgers. Igor was afraid to spoil the ingredients. He reasoned, "It was easy with real meat—you just cut a piece and fry it with oil. But now I am supposed to create 'meat' from carrots, and without a cow?" He saw me preparing live garden burgers dozens of times but he was certain that it was too complicated for him. One day we had an emergency situation when too many people showed up for a catered raw-food dinner. I was busy preparing soup. Somebody had to prepare garden burgers, and Igor didn't have a choice. So he did it! Even before I finished making soup he was done. Since that day I have never made another live garden burger myself because Igor took over this task. Now in my family we call this dish "Igorburger."

Igor enjoyed preparing raw food more and more. He created many of his own recipes. His Russian Borodinsky crackers are popular all over the world (also called "Igor's Crackers" and found under that name in this book). In Iceland Igor demonstrated how to prepare a raw sandwich. He put live garden burgers on crackers and decorated them with green leaves and tomatoes. When people tried his raw sandwiches they were amazed at how delicious they were. One woman exclaimed: "This sandwich is worth living for!"

In this chapter I share important tips for preparing gourmet dishes through the transitional stage of your raw-food life. I don't think anybody needs my recommendations for their further stages because after several months of living on a raw-food diet, most people feel comfortable preparing their own meals.

Many ingredients in cooked dishes always have the same standard taste. For example, sugar always tastes like sugar, flour like flour, and salt is always salt. In raw-food cuisine, no two lemons are alike. One is bigger and has more juice; the other one has thicker skin and is less sour. Cooked corn, cooked zucchini, cooked peas, and other cooked vegetables taste almost the same and require at least the addition of oil and salt. By comparison, raw corn, zucchini, peas, and other raw vegetables all have their own unique tastes that are impossible to confuse.

For this reason, when preparing a raw dish, following a recipe doesn't guarantee a delicious result. You need to always adjust the final taste. When I prepare a raw dish I use recipes only as ideas or general guidelines. For adjusting the final taste I use the "method of five tastes." The rule is to have an element of each flavor in every dish. These five tastes are: *sweet, sour, salty, spicy,* and *bitter.* When you learn to balance the five tastes, your food will stimulate different groups of taste buds, thus making the food delicious.

In nature, all fruits and vegetables already have a balanced bouquet of tastes. However, the taste buds in our mouth have been altered from years of eating cooked food filled with condiments. That is why we are unable to sense all of the delicate natural flavors in raw fruits and vegetables while eating cooked food. As our taste buds recover during the transition time to a raw-food diet, we begin enjoying simpler foods.

When you attempt to un-cook a delicious meal, make sure that all five flavors are present in the final bouquet—that not even one is missing. People who have been preparing raw gourmet meals every day for many months can definitely tell if one or two ingredients are missing by just tasting the food once or twice. Others have to taste freshly made meals five times, asking each time very simple questions: "Is it spicy enough? Is it salty enough? Is it sweet enough? Is it sour enough? Is it bitter enough?" The five tastes don't have to be strong but just enough for a particular dish. For example, the strongest tastes in a garden burger should be sweet, spicy, and salty with only a touch of sour and bitter, but all five have to be present. Otherwise the garden burger will taste bland.

Usually, when you prepare a dish and go through your first round of five-spoon tasting, two or three tastes are missing. Add ingredients for the missing tastes, mix again, and start five-spoon tasting once more. Continue until the five major tastes are balanced into a nice bouquet. I call this process "adjusting the taste." In the beginning adjusting can take a long time. Don't be discouraged; your pace will speed up with practice. At the same time your raw food will become unbeatable.

The following is a list of suggested ingredients for the five taste groups. Please be creative, as this is only a fraction of what is available on planet Earth. Many plants possess a variety of tastes but have one or two that are dominant. Also, please apply common sense and don't add vanilla to the soup or garlic to the torte.

For a sour taste add: lemons, cranberries, rhubarb, lemon grass, sour grass, sorrel, tomatoes, sauerkraut, nut or seed yogurt, or apple cider vinegar.

For a sweet taste add: dried fruit such as figs, dates, prunes, raisins; fresh fruits such as ripe banana, mango, peach, pear; apple juice, orange juice, raw agave nectar, raw honey, or fresh stevia leaves.

For spicy taste add: garlic or onion shoots, cloves, or bulbs, ginger, mustard greens or seeds, radish, horseradish, cayenne pepper, wasabi, seaweed, and/or herbs—fresh or dry—such as basil, dill, cilantro, rosemary, cinnamon, nutmeg, vanilla, and peppermint.

For salty taste add: celery, cilantro, dill, parsley, or sea vegetables such as dulse, kelp, nori, arame, or Celtic sea salt.

For bitter taste add: parsley, celery tops, endive, garlic, onion, dandelion, bay leaf, sage, poultry seasoning, or cayenne pepper.

I believe that skillfully prepared raw-food dishes are comparable to the most sophisticated cooked recipes, and in many cases raw-food dishes taste better. I personally stopped telling people that my food was raw a long time ago, beginning with the wedding that I was invited to cater. The couple to be married didn't ask for a raw wedding and due to my desire to be hired, I didn't push to clarify. However, I was confident that I could satisfy their palates whether they wanted raw or cooked food for their reception. I enjoyed preparing and decorating the three-tier raw wedding cake. I made lots of beautiful finger foods, colorful refreshments, a big salad with a variety of dressings, and nut patties. I remember how my daughter and I spent several hours drawing lines on those patties, making them look like real barbecued burgers.

Then the reception began. There were about fifty guests, and no one noticed anything unusual for about an hour. Then people started having questions and called the chef (me) to the dining hall. When I came out they asked me, "Is this Russian cuisine? What kind of herbs did you use in everything? Your food is so good, but we've never tasted anything like it!"

I looked at this group of fifty people and suddenly realized that knowing all the food was raw would be a shock to them. They looked at me quizzically. I asked them, "Would you like to come into the kitchen? I'll show you how I made it."

My kitchen space filled with many curious guests, and I prepared two dishes very quickly in front of them: nut meat pâté and a candy ball. All the guests were amazed by how speedy, simple, and tasty the results were. Now they forgot all about the bride and the groom and began asking questions. Women were grabbing pens out of their husband's pockets and scribbling on napkins, on each other's shoulders, asking, "How much lemon did you say?" One chubby-looking man wanted to know, "Can you teach my wife how to make this food?" Later that week I held a huge class that was filled with many guests from this wedding.

Over many years of eating raw food, everyone in my family has learned how to quickly fix delicious meals. Based on our experience, we have developed simple techniques that we successfully teach to thousands of other raw-fooders. Following are five formulas that are incredibly simple, almost primitive. They enable anyone to prepare tasty, quick, easy, and inexpensive raw gourmet meals.

Basic Formula for Delicious Soup

The base

Five flavors

Something to float (for example, grated carrot or other root, chunks of avocado or some vegetable, chopped parsley or other herbs)

The base for the soup is always the same:

1 cup water

1 stalk celery

1 tablespoon olive oil

Mix everything in the blender except the floating chunks; add them afterwards. I use this simple formula for any gourmet soup that I prepare.

Yield: 2 cups of soup

Basic Formula for Delicious Nut Burgers

1 cup any nuts

1 cup any vegetables

1 tablespoon oil to make it stick together

Five flavors

Mix in a food processor.

Note: If you want a heavier burger, put more nuts. For a lighter burger, use more vegetables.

Yield: 2 cups of burger pâté

Basic Formula for Delicious Candy or Cake Dough

1 cup any nuts

1 cup any dried fruits

1 tablespoon oil to make it stick together

Spices (optional)

Mix in a food processor. Roll candies or use as crust layers for the cake.

Yield: 2 cups of delicious dough

Formula for Delicious Dressing

1/2 cup water

2 tablespoons olive oil

Five strong flavors

Blend well.

Yield: 3/4 cup of delicious dressing

Basic Formula for Delicious Nut or Seed Milk

1/2 cup any nuts or seeds, soaked in water overnight and drained

1 cup water

1 tablespoon sweetener (optional)

Blend well and strain through a nut milk bag. For "skim" milk use more water.

I LOVE YOU NO MATTER WHAT YOU EAT

"A man may well bring a horse to the water, but he cannot make him drink."

—John Heywood, *Proverbs*

Once at my workshop I asked my audience a question: *"What emotions do you feel when someone tells you what to do?"*

Most of us have probably been given unsolicited advice countless times, beginning from childhood. Remember when you were a kid and your mom or your dad said, "You're running around in the streets too much, you really need to read more books"? Try recalling how you felt in such a situation. Did you immediately feel drawn to books? Did you say, "Oh, thank you, Dad, I'll go and read right now!"? Chances are you felt rebellious and resentful, and the last thing you wanted to do was pick up a book, sit down, and read. Or recall a time when a friend said to you something along the lines of, "You need to start jogging. You're getting fat." Or, "You should cut off those awful dreadlocks." Or, "You really should stop smoking. You have children." What was your reaction? Did these suggestions help you? Probably not. Following are some of my students' responses to other people's "helpful suggestions."

Nancy: I would breathe a little smile, but of course I wouldn't do it.

Mike: I'd get angry and resentful.

Dorothy: I would feel defensive, and I hate that feeling.

Bryan: I'd feel really sarcastic.

Jane: I would feel hurt, insulted, angry, and offended.

Whitney: I wouldn't do it, because it's not their choice. I'd have resistance.

George: I'd just smile and ignore.

Cynthia: I hate being forced and I'd have to start being dishonest.

Wendy: I want to please. I want to do what they ask me to do, but then I'll be secretive about it and be resentful.

Seth: I'd want to kill that person!

Carla: I would feel a wave of depression take a hold of me, probably for a long time.

Sam: When they think I should change something, I won't do it even if I know it's right, but I'll get mad that I know it's right and I'm not doing it.

Ryan: I would feel inferior and put down.

Linda: I would feel as if they were trying to control me and I would rebel.

As you may see, when someone tells us that he or she knows what is good for us, we tend to feel angry and upset. We feel annoyed, negative, and we shut them and their advice out. We feel attacked, hurt, and uncomfortable.

That is precisely how our friends and family would feel when we tried advising them to eat more raw food. Similarly, the announcement of a family member becoming a raw-fooder can be frightening news for the rest of the family. Cooked food is what most of us know and consider normal; it's what is expected in our culture. Do we really want those we love to feel rebellious, negative, shut off, controlled, or angry? This is exactly how they are likely to feel if we tell them one day, "I'm going to be raw now, so don't eat that crap in front of me! Just the look of it makes me sick!"

I recommend doing exactly the opposite. When you decide to become a raw-fooder, talk to your family. Explain to them, "You know, darling, this is not about you. Eating raw food is the choice I am making for myself. I'm not asking you to eat raw food. It's really okay with me that you continue to eat your favorite steak. I love you the way you are. It's me who's trying to change. It's not about you. I don't expect you to follow me, to be interested, or even to try my food." When you talk to your family in this manner, you may notice how they will sigh with relief.

Sometimes we may make those we love feel uncomfortable even without words. Some of us throw certain glances that convey the same meaning as the disapproving words. For example, a woman in one of my classes said to me, "My family is angry with my raw-foodism even though I never pushed anybody to eat raw food. My husband has been vegan for thirty years. My son is twelve. They always ask me to prepare cooked meals. When I cook food for them I go off my raw-food diet. I don't feel supported. My son makes all kinds of jokes about me having to eat my raw cake with a spoon."

I said to her, "You might be doing something that irritates them that you're not aware of. Just watch yourself, and catch those moments. Don't watch others. Watch and see what you are doing to antagonize your family."

The next week she came to class and said, "Yeah. I caught myself several times poking little pins in certain painful places. I'd say something hurtful or look disgusted or put out. I changed my attitude toward my family, and they, in turn, shifted towards me and it only took one week. When I started accepting them, then they accepted me back. Now my husband is making juice for me in the morning and even bringing it to me in bed. He says, 'Honey, I want you to stay on raw food.' Suddenly my house has become a peaceful place, and my son is willing to try everything I make."

I am making my living by teaching raw-food classes, and I have been on a 100% raw-food diet for many years. But twenty years ago when I was still eating a traditional diet, I had a friend who was a raw-foodist. I remember how annoyed I would get by his comments. Once, my older son Stephan was in the hospital with a minor surgery. My raw-food friend was critical about me allowing this to happen. Today, I feel embarrassed when I recall how furious I was towards my friend for his advice. I wasn't ready then.

Another example is my friend Tina from Denver. She had a serious health problem. For many months she had to go to the hospital to undergo a procedure that was extremely painful for her. When we came to visit, she saw what Igor and I were eating and she became interested. She asked, "Can you show me how to prepare this food? I'm willing to try because I have surgery (a colostomy) scheduled in two weeks which I would rather not do." Within a matter of days, she started feeling better and avoided the surgery. Tina understood that for her, there were only two choices: raw food, no surgery, life and health; or cooked food, surgery, and eventually death. Tina chose life. At the time of our visit, Tina's four children were major junk-food eaters, and her husband enjoyed vodka, steak, pork chops, and pig's fat, which he used as if it were bologna. Tina did not tell her family that she was going raw. She kept cooking for them as she always had. She said, "I'm going to keep it quiet." I agreed with her and said, "Don't even mention it to them. Don't irritate them. Let them just leave you alone. Tell your family that you don't expect them to do anything." Tina didn't mention her diet change to them.

One year passed. We were driving through Denver again and we stopped by. I saw Tina's husband, Sam, and he looked dramatically different. I said, "Sam, what's happening? You've changed." He replied with a grin, "I became 100% raw one month ago. The children are raw, too."

I was shocked. "What happened?"

Sam told me the story of why he became raw. He said that one day, about a month ago, he went to pick up Tina at work. He arrived a little early and sat down within view of her desk to wait. He noticed that his wife was so beautiful. He saw the customers flirting with his wife. He was looking at her through new eyes. He saw how she'd become so healthy, sexy, and attractive. All of a sudden he felt inadequate. He said, "I ran to the restroom and I looked at myself in a mirror. I saw puffs under my eyes and a red face and gray hairs sticking out all over. I opened my shirt, and I looked at the blemishes all over my chest. I thought, nobody is going to flirt with me!" Sam told me that he realized Tina had been getting healthy and beautiful and he was just aging. Sam decided to make a change so he could keep up with his wife. He said, "On the way back home I begged her to help me become raw like her."

Tina was happy to help her husband. She told me that as soon as Sam adopted a raw-food diet, the children said they wanted to eat raw food too! Her daughter became thin and beautiful and was now auditioning for a local theater. Everything in this family's life was transforming in a wonderful way. Tina said that she felt a call from God, and things happened like never before in their life. Tina is a very wise woman. She didn't preach to her family about eating raw food. She made her food and enjoyed it without putting any expectations on her relatives. Her body healed and her family observed the changes. Because of her good example, her family made the choice to follow.

I can recall many similar examples that show the importance of living in peace with people who eat cooked food. When we don't understand how important this is, we can ruin the peace around ourselves and turn it into war. We can make people irritated by raw food. At the same time, we can make a conscious choice to live in peace with those around us. Then the miracles can happen. We have no right to control others. We have no right to expect other people to change when they are not ready. In contrast, our duty is to explain to others that we don't expect them to change.

That doesn't mean that there won't be any more family dinners. Why not? You may tell your partner, "Honey, let's have a family dinner. You may bring your pork chops and I'll bring my stuffed bell pepper. We'll talk about our day and we'll enjoy our time together." After all, family is about love. Family is not about food. When loved ones know that we do not expect anything from them, they can relax around us. They can support us without feeling pressured to change. We have made a choice for ourselves for serious reasons. We made the right choice for us, though perhaps it is not the right choice for everyone.

However, when I first went on a raw-food diet I did just the opposite of my advice to you. I went around telling everyone to go on raw food. For a while I was chasing overweight ladies in Safeway, trying to explain to them how easy it is to lose weight. I was so excited about the healthy changes my family was experiencing, I got carried away. I made a lot of enemies before I understood that people need to find their own ways and decide their own paths.

When we respect other people's rights, we may ask for support from our loved ones. We need to be sincere and not afraid to tell them, "My darling, please help me. I need support. I need to eat raw food for my health, because when I eat cooked food I feel as if I'm falling apart. When I eat raw food, I feel more energy and I have more love for you. Please help me. I don't need you to be raw. I have an idea. Instead of buying me chocolates on Sunday, will you buy me a ripe mango? Or any exotic fruit would be a great pleasure for me. I so appreciate your thoughtfulness. It would be so helpful to me if you'd keep those cookies that we have on the living room table in your truck so that I can't eat them in a moment of weakness. I appreciate your support so much."

Don't be afraid to be vulnerable and tell your family and close friends, "Listen, I need your help. It is important for me and my health now that I go on raw food. Without your help I cannot do it. Support me; don't offer me any cooked food. You may eat absolutely whatever you want but don't offer it to me, please." To ask for support is different than advising them to go on a raw-food diet. People love to be supportive, because we usually have love in our families and among friends.

Millie is a good example. When Millie was diagnosed with breast cancer, she began eating raw food. Her whole family (three adult sons along with her husband) were hostile and just hated the word "raw." Then Millie attended the 12 Steps to Raw Foods workshop.

With Step Four in mind, she went through and rearranged her communication with her family. I received an email from her some weeks after the class. She wrote, "My husband is growing proud of me! Everything is working out miraculously. My family now understands that I need support." She made it clear to her family that she needed their support to heal her cancer; and since she didn't demand that they eat raw food, there was no pressure on them. At the same time, they were glad to help her in any way they could.

No matter how we would love the rest of the family to benefit from eating raw food, we can control only one person in the world—ourselves. It is not our business to control our children or our parents, even if they are dying from cancer. I learned my lesson when my mother was dying from bone cancer, and I flew all the way to Russia to put her on a raw-food diet so she would survive. I was working very hard, going to the farmers' market, buying vegetables and juicing them all day long. On the third day, as soon as I left for the market, my mother whispered to my brother, "Son, can you make me some scrambled eggs? I'm starving!" When I returned, my mother's room was filled with the smell of scrambled eggs. My brother said, "I don't want to lie to you. She asked for it." In that moment I realized how cruel it was for me to put pressure on my poor mother. If she was not really ready, then my persistence only caused her more suffering. We have already discussed how we feel when someone tells us something we are not ready for.

I know one young man from Seattle who told me that he felt sorry for his mother, who suffered from tremendous pain. He told me that he and his mother were closest friends in the world. He confided, "I wish she would go on raw food so she wouldn't have to suffer."

I asked him, "Do you know that you might make her suffer even more through her feeling that she is not meeting your expectation?"

He said, "I never thought of that." After he gave it some thought, he came home and told his mother, "You know, it's okay with me if you're not going to try my diet." In a few days he called me back and reported, "A miracle happened—Mom wants to try my food!"

When people aren't forced to change their diet and feel safe and un-judged about what they eat, it's often the case that they suddenly want to improve their eating habits. If we learn how to live in peace with people who eat cooked food, we are more likely to receive support instead of opposition.

I met people who started pushing others onto raw food even before they tried it themselves—like Linda. After Linda visited just one raw-food class she demanded her friend Jim to go on a raw-food diet. She came to the next class and complained that Jim didn't support her. Somehow she managed to drag Jim to my last class. By then, he had already developed such strong prejudice and resistance towards raw foods that he sat in the farthest corner of the classroom. However, after listening to the lecture, Jim became very interested. Two months later Jim called me and said that he had been staying on the raw diet for the past two months, but Linda found it challenging and went back to eating cooked food. Ironically, Jim began dating another woman that he met at the raw-food potluck.

When you prepare your raw lunch or dinner that you are planning to eat with your family, don't let your plate consist of just a bunch of sprouts. Your family might feel sorry for you, thinking that you are deprived of pleasures. Instead, prepare yourself a nice-looking gourmet dish. Later, your loved ones will be drawn to try some of your food because it looks so attractive. When they taste your raw creation, they might comment, "It's not bad."

What about the children in your house that you need to prepare meals for? In many cases, we have already hooked our children on cooked foods, and that is why we have to be patient with them. In some cases it is better to slowly increase the ratio of raw food to cooked food. I recommend that everyone always have plenty of raw fruits and vegetables handy for snacks. Learn how to make raw ice creams, nut milks, nut-milk shakes, smoothies, live candies, cakes, and other kid-friendly foods. Show your children that raw food can be enjoyable. Invite them to prepare raw food together. Buy them a cheap blender at a garage sale. But most importantly, be a good example and don't make a big fuss about raw foods. Remember, kids learn by watching others. Let them see harmony and love around the table.

I am often asked how not to insult relatives who use food to show their love. If their food is refused, they may feel rejected and disrespected. In response to this question, I say, "The next time we meet I will bring a bottle of vodka, and if you don't drink it with me right away, while standing up with a toast to health, you will dis-respect me as a native Russian." In this situation I assume that most of you would have no problem finding a way of declining my offer without insulting me or conveying disrespect. If you still feel con-fused, here are some more tips on saying "No" without offending anyone.

If people bring us food as a sign of their love, then showing our sincere appreciation for their care would make them most happy. According to a wonderful system called the "Nonviolent Commu-nication Process,"[1] the best way we can demonstrate our appreciation is by expressing our sincere gratitude and describing our true feelings.

For example, John's aunt brought him an apple pie that used to be his favorite dessert. She made it herself. Below are two possible scenarios.

Scenario 1.

John: "What is this? Oh no, I cannot have this! It is cooked and loaded with sugar. I don't eat this food anymore, don't you know that?! People who eat such stuff get sick. Why? Because cooked dough plugs their bowels. It's like eating glue! I don't want to offend you, but I must speak the truth. Why are you crying, Auntie?"

Scenario 2.

John: "What is this, Auntie? Oh, that is your famous apple pie! I am so deeply touched by your loving care. You must have spent so much money and time in order to please me. I feel so special. Thank you so much! Please come in, sit down, I am looking forward to sharing with you about the latest change in my diet. I feel a lot more energy. Next time you need help in your yard I can handle a lot more work. Would you like to try some almond milk? I am so glad you came."

While the conversation in the first scenario would most likely leave a bitter trace in the memories of both people, the sincere appreciation of the second scenario allows John to explain his motives to his aunt without upsetting her. Since John's aunt cares to please him with his favorite treat, she definitely loves John and would be delighted to discover that her nephew is making positive changes in his life.

When I went to Russia and refused the traditional Russian food, my relatives felt offended for a while, but then when they noticed how important raw food is for me and my health, they weren't upset anymore. I showed them pictures of myself before adopting a raw-food diet. They confirmed that I looked better on "that rabbit diet" than I had before. They never knew that I could look so good. If there is a loving atmosphere in the family, we can always find appropriate words to explain our position and be heard. Human beings have a curious nature and can easily be inspired. I have noticed that people enjoy finding their own answers to their questions. Perhaps the biggest way we can help others is by raising their curiosity. After all, we cannot change others. The only person I can really transform is myself. However, I have unlimited power over myself; and I see infinite possibilities to better myself. If every one of us keeps improving individually, together we can change the world.

Step 5

AVOIDING TEMPTATIONS

"It is not the mountains that we conquer, but ourselves."

—Sir Edmund Hillary

According to the *Merriam-Webster Online Dictionary*, the word "temptation" means "the desire to have or do something that you know you should *avoid*."[1] (Emphasis added.) The meaning of "temptation" seems to be paradoxical: we strongly desire something that is bad for us. How can such a phenomenon even be possible?

Let us observe the temptation to eat unhealthy foods. Most people are aware that eating poorly may, eventually, result in pain, disease, and even premature death. These consequences sound awful, don't they? Then what compels so many of us to deliberately consume various unhealthy foods? The secret is in those brief but instant pleasures that come with eating certain dishes, while the consequences happen in the long run, often after many years.

Temptations are possibly humans' foremost challenge in life. However illusory, temptations possess an enormous power over many people. It's no wonder that many world religions consider temptations to come from the devil. I witnessed countless times how the sight of but one bite of some nostalgic food caused people to cross out their many months of work towards eating healthy.

Since the vast majority of people in the world live on predominantly cooked foods, adopting a raw-food lifestyle always presents a challenge shaped in a multitude of temptations. These enticements can quickly overturn one's plans for healthy eating if not properly approached. Based on many years of personal observations and helping people stay on a raw-food diet, I strongly believe that we cannot fight temptations by sheer will power. For that reason I have developed a strategy that has helped me, as well as many other people.

Many psychologists consider the first and most important step in overcoming temptations to be determining the main long-term goal of any pursuit. Therefore, you need to figure out what your main goal in adopting a raw-food diet is. Perhaps you have many targets, such as losing weight, gaining more energy, healing a certain illness, and so forth. However, research clearly demonstrates that when you choose one *main* long-term goal, you will concentrate all your attention on attaining this particular purpose, and as a result you will be able to decline momentary pleasures more easily.[2]

In addition, I recommend that you analyze on a deeper level your motives to eat healthy and to spell out your most inspiring purpose for becoming a raw-foodist that will keep motivating you for years and enable you to overcome all temptations along your way.

The trouble with temptations is that they distract us from conscious living. Our existence is penetrated with cruel enticements. Some of them are so powerful that we often confuse temptations with our major goals in life. For example, I have met many people who sincerely believed that their life purpose was to own a nice TV, to party as much as possible, and/or to possess a lot of money. To me, all those things are merely big temptations, while the true purpose of life is a spiritual idea—something that everyone is destined to discover on his or her own. I believe that everyone has a true mission in life and that this mission is connected with helping other people. For me, discovering the purpose of life is *the most* precious gift for every human. When we have a purpose, we know which direction to follow in life, and as we move towards the focal goal, we feel happy and fulfilled. On the contrary, if we haven't found our life mission yet, we keep walking in place and begin feeling useless and depressed.

Having a healthy body can be instrumental in both finding and fulfilling one's life mission; otherwise instead of helping others, we will be the ones in need of help. Our body, our psyche, and our spirit are the only instruments we have for living; without them we cannot perform any actions and cannot accomplish any goals. Therefore, if we possess the best possible health attainable, our life mission can be performed better. People who have a chance to improve their health through better eating might discover benefits of much greater value than merely good physical health.

Considering all of this reasoning, I encourage you to now think of all the possible missions that you are going to accomplish by following a healthy lifestyle and choose one purpose as your most important target. I would like to clarify that "becoming a raw-foodist" is not a *goal*, but rather a *means* for reaching a *goal*. Write your *main goal* down. Read it out loud. Does your *main goal* sound exciting to you? I recommend that you learn your *main goal* by heart and repeat it as an affirmation whenever you need support. I hope this goal will provide you with strength, support, and inspiration for many years.

I would like to share with you another tactic useful for overcoming temptations. The following exercise helps you identify places and times in your life where you need to be alert and ready for a challenge. List in a column all possible temptations that might interfere with attaining your *main goal*. Try to remember all the places where you have been tempted in the last couple of weeks and list them all, even if you have to continue for several pages. To help you recognize your possible temptations, I offer some of the examples listed by students in my workshops:

- the coffee smell at the bookstore
- lunch break at work
- vending machines in the lobby
- commercials
- my friends eating chocolate
- mom's cooking
- returning from work after 5 p.m. hungry
- free samples in the store
- free candy at my bank
- passing a drive-thru on the way home
- being inside a gas station
- participating in a party
- popcorn at the movie theater
- being the only raw-foodist in my home

Considering the potentially immense power of each tiny temptation, you want to be prepared to be "attacked" at any time. By all means, try to avoid temptations whenever possible. Take all tempting cooked foods out of your house, office, and car. Don't leave a hidden stash of your favorite cooked food in the house, because the thought of it will be chasing you until you eat this food, making it hard for you to relax or concentrate on your work. When we are hungry, angry, lonely, or depressed, we often think that eating our favorite food will help numb our feelings.

Try avoiding advertisements at least for several months. When advertisers promote eating junk food, they portray a good time where everyone is smiling. The advertisers leave out the negative consequences of unhealthy eating, such as sickness, becoming overweight, or depression. Most of the ads connect cooked food to happy social events. The advertisers attempt to create an image suggesting that if we eat the product advertised, we'll be as happy and fulfilled as the people appear in the ad. We all know the ad is staged and the people are actors, but we still crave the food and the *feeling* in the ad.

Now write your strategies next to each temptation listed. Try to substitute temptations with pleasant activities, rather than simply deleting tempting actions from your life (which isn't always possible anyway). Prepare specific strategies for the enticements you cannot avoid. Be realistic and don't place much of your hope on your will power. Following are various strategies used by some of my students:

- Coffee smell at the bookstore: *I will order books online.*
- Lunch break at work: *I will always bring a big, delicious raw lunch to work.*
- Vending machines in the lobby: *I will recite a poem while passing it.*
- Commercials on TV: *I will watch only rental movies.*
- Commercials in magazines: *I will ask someone to remove pages with ads before reading a magazine myself or read a book instead.*
- My friends eating chocolate: *I will eat a fruit at the same time or I will say affirmations.*

- Mom's cooking: *I will teach mom raw dishes, buy her a blender.*
- Returning from work after 5 p.m.: *I will put on nice music.*
- Free samples in the store: *I will stuff my mouth with raisins.*
- Free candy at my bank: *I will use drive-thru banking.*
- Passing a drive-thru on a way home: *I will choose another route home.*
- Being inside a gas station: *I will pay outside with a credit card.*
- Participating in a party: *I will excuse myself now. When I feel stronger I will bring my own dish to the party.*
- Popcorn at the movie theater: *I will bring a bag of sliced fruits and veggies.*
- Being the only raw-foodist in my home: *I will designate a part of our kitchen as a temptation-free zone.*

Denying ourselves little pleasures can be frustrating, especially in the beginning. Try to concentrate on the positive side of your transformation to raw-food eating. Remind yourself often that while you choose to miss a party, you are gaining qualities of much greater value than the quick pleasure of eating. While eating healthy, you are constantly receiving the precious gifts of good health in many different forms: vibrant energy, clarity of mind, good-looking skin, sweet breath, improved vision, and countless more. Most importantly, you are coming closer and closer to your *main goal.*

Research has demonstrated that if we keep avoiding daily temptations, we eventually develop an automatic (subconscious) response to them and stop noticing temptations altogether.[3]

When you have built some resistance to temptations, you may go out to restaurants alone or better yet, with a friend. You may bring your own dressing and some raw crackers or little sprouted seeds to put on top of the salad.

To make going out easier and more enjoyable, I recommend using a "restaurant card." My friend Jonathan Weber invented this card a long time ago and it has since served thousands of raw-fooders. You can make your "restaurant card" approximately the size of a business card. Present it to a waitress when she takes your order. This card saves me unnecessary complications when I go out to eat. Instead of lengthy explanations of what I can or cannot eat, I simply hand my card to the waitress. My experience has shown that most restaurant chefs find this approach to be helpful and appreciate a chance to be creative. Thanks to using my "restaurant card," my dishes always reach my table attractive and delicious. Print many of these cards and give them away to all your friends. When waitresses report the growing number of requests for raw foods to their managers, raw-food dishes will appear on the menus of many more restaurants.

Jonathan's Card

I EAT ONLY RAW, UNCOOKED FOODS
I would like a salad or vegetable plate with only fresh, uncooked items:

lettuce	*tomato*	*avocado*	*carrot*
zucchini	*sprouts*	*cucumber*	*celery*
broccoli	*scallions*	*radish*	*onion*
cauliflower	*parsley*	*cabbage*	*kale*
spinach	*cilantro*	*bell pepper*	*beets*
mushrooms	*bok choy*	*arugula*	*chard*

Thank you for your creative effort!

After a couple of months of staying on a raw-food diet and deliberately handling your temptations, you will notice that you stop paying attention to restaurants and any cooked food in general. You might also get the false impression that your attraction to cooked food has disappeared, and you may *feel tempted* to eat or try small pieces of cooked food once in a while. That is probably the most deceptive enticement of all. I have seen many people unwittingly terminate their raw-food diet with one such bite. I recommend that you try to forget about cooked delicacies altogether and instead keep cherishing and approaching your *main goal.*

Step 6

GETTING SUPPORT

"Man is a child of his environment."

—Shinichi Suzuki

Humans have been challenged by temptations since the beginning of time, or perhaps since they experienced their first pleasures. The ancient Greek poet Homer created a perfect metaphor for temptation—the Sirens. In Greek mythology, the Siren is a creature with the head of a female and the body of a bird, and it lives on small rocky islands. With the irresistible charm of their songs the Sirens lured mariners to their destruction on the rocks surrounding their islands. In his epic poem *The Odyssey*, Homer described how the main character Odysseus conquered the Sirens (temptations) using his intelligence and the support of his crew. Forewarned of the Sirens' seductive musical reputation, Odysseus saved his ships from the fatal songs. When they passed the islands of the Sirens, he had the sailors stuff their ears with wax. Odysseus ordered his crew to tie him to the mast, for he wanted to hear the beautiful singing. When Odysseus's ship approached, the Sirens began to sing, their words even more enticing than their melody. They were promising to give knowledge to every man who came to them, along with ripe wisdom and a quickening of the spirit. Odysseus' heart ran with longing, but the ropes held him, and the ship quickly sailed to safe waters.[1]

I find this story meaningful. I doubt that Odysseus would have stayed on the ship had he not been tied to the mast. Without the tight ropes, he would have followed the Sirens and died, as everybody else had before him. He wouldn't have been able to stand the temptation by will power alone. I assume that Odysseus had unusually strong will power, since he was portrayed as a hero in a poem. Yet he ordered his sailors to tie him down. This is an important message for all of us: to conquer temptation, being a hero is not enough. One also has to be wise and not afraid to ask for help. At certain times, when we encounter an unusually strong temptation, we should seek help from outside ourselves, from another person or a group of people. We must "tie ourselves to the mast" ahead of time, before "passing the islands of the Sirens." That is, we must seek support to avoid especially strong temptations.

I recommend that you get all the support you possibly can. Following are several ideas any beginner can use to organize support.

Go to raw-food potlucks or better yet, open your own house to weekly or monthly raw-food potlucks. You will have to do some cleaning, spend some time and energy, but the support that you will gain is invaluable. The two main benefits of a potluck are that it is free and everyone is challenged to prepare, decorate, and serve a dish. In my hometown of Ashland, Oregon, we have several ongoing small potlucks in different homes, and once a month we have a large potluck, open to all people.

Another popular way of supporting yourself is organizing a weekly "soup and salad dinner for five dollars." Buy any produce on sale, prepare a large bowl of soup, cut up some veggies, and make a jug of dressing. Then invite people from your local community to stop by and have dinner at your place. Put flyers up at the local health food store or place an announcement in the newspaper. You may do it once a week at a certain time, say 5–7 p.m. on Wednesdays. Put a jar for donations on the table. This event has many benefits over potlucks: people don't have to worry about preparing food, they have a social environment without having to tip a waiter, it is reasonably priced, they could always afford to bring a friend, and the host makes a little cash. We have kept this event going in Ashland very successfully for long periods of time.

Begin teaching classes about raw food. If you don't want to teach the theory, you can teach food preparation. After only two weeks on a raw-food diet, you will be capable of making at least a couple of dishes, maybe almond milk, live soup, salad dressing, etc. Share with others how to prepare these basic dishes. You could charge money or teach for free, because remember, you're doing it for the sake of support.

Subscribe to raw-food magazines.* They usually contain the freshest news and most current ideas on many important raw-food issues. There are so many different writers sharing their encouragement, personal experiences, and viewpoints. Raw-food magazines give incredible support. I always read them cover to cover.

Search the Internet. There are many websites devoted to living foods. Many of them have personal ads, bulletin boards, and chat rooms where you can meet a raw buddy or find raw-food communities near you. Following is a list of some popular websites:

- http://www.goneraw.com

Living Nutrition magazine, published in California. More information at: www.livingnutrition.com. *Get Fresh! Magazine*, published in the United Kingdom. More information at: http://www.fresh-network.com/getfresh/index.htm.

- http://www.living-foods.net
- http://www.rawfamily.com
- http://www.rawlivingfoodresources.com
- http://www.naturesrawenergy.com
- http://www.treeoflife.nu
- http://www.arnoldsway.com
- http://www.RawRawGirls.com
- http://www.rawfoodtalk.com

I recommend that you sign up for a couple of e-newsletters. Following are the websites where you may find some of the most helpful newsletters:

- http://www.arnoldsway.com
- http://www.TheGardenDiet.com
- http://www.rawfamily.com
- http://www.alokhealth.com
- http://www.chidiet.com

Go to raw food lectures, not only to listen to the speaker but also to communicate with other attendees—I am not sure which is more important! For this reason, I favor going to raw-food festivals, where for one flat fee you can listen to many distinguished speakers and share valuable conversations with hundreds or thousands of other participants, enjoy gourmet meals together, and find new friends with similar life interests or sometimes with the same health issues. Following is a list of several popular raw-food events:

- Vibrant Living Expo, annual, California, USA. For more details, call: 707-964-2420 or visit: www.RawFoodChef.com.
- Raw Spirit Retreat, annual, Oregon, USA. For more details, call 503-650-4447.

- The Fresh Festival, annual, United Kingdom. For more details visit: http://www.fresh-network.com/festival/index.htm.
- Raw World: International Festival of Raw Food Enthusiasts, annual, Costa Rica. For more details visit: www.rawworld.org.
- Raw Spirit Festival, annual, Arizona, USA. For more details, call: 928-708-0784; 928-284-0759 and 928-776-1497.

To create a more supportive environment around you, maintain close physical proximity to people and groups that are associated with your *main goal*, as well as with staying on a healthy diet. For example, signing up with your local jogging club will bring you in touch with runners who are also interested in health; therefore they will indirectly provide support for you. You may become involved in activities with groups of people who have related or similar interests. They might reinforce your motivations and provide an environment that has little or no temptations. Following is a list of various ideas from my students:

- Become a member of the local YMCA.
- Visit the farmers' market weekly.
- Become a member of a local CSA coop (Community-Supported Agriculture).
- Participate in local EarthSave groups.
- Travel to a raw-food festival once a year.
- Grow an organic garden in the back yard.
- Get a pass to a swimming pool.
- Sign up at a fitness club.
- Participate in a massage workshop.
- Get involved in U-pick activities at local organic orchards.
- Become involved in vegan potlucks.

When staying on a raw-food diet without support, you may feel that you are the only raw-fooder in the whole world and even that you are weird. At the same time, the support of even one person can make you feel as though half of the world has already adopted this way of eating. Keep in mind that by staying on raw foods, you *too* are providing support for others.

Step 7

GRATITUDE AND FORGIVENESS

"Gratitude is not only the greatest of virtues, but the parent of all others."

—Cicero

When we adopt a raw-food lifestyle, we may feel deprived of our habitual pleasures, especially when we watch others enjoying cooked delicacies that used to be our own favorites. Being hungry, angry, lonely, or depressed at that moment could add even more frustration to our feelings of misery. I would like to share with you a method that can help eliminate feelings of deprivation from your life forever.

We all have different perspectives on life. Some of us feel that life is becoming increasingly more frustrating, especially considering all the natural cataclysms and political challenges. At the same time, others view life as a totally beautiful and enjoyable experience. Initially, I thought that our opinions on the fairness of life depended on the level of our material wealth. Later, I met some poor people who were content with their lives and wealthy persons who were deeply upset about their lives. While watching many people caught in a material pursuit (including myself), I developed a strong interest in the true origins of people's contentment in life. I came to the conclusion that there are two opposite perspectives on life: the materialistic perspective and the grateful perspective.

The materialistic approach to life guarantees discontentment and frustration, as there is no objective limit to the acquisition of personal possessions. There is no constant measure that could be marked as "enough." At the same time, only the very basic possessions that satisfy our essential needs such as food, clothes, and shelter can bring us a sensible feeling of contentment. The majority of items beyond the basic needs convey very little enjoyment to their possessor.

Contrary to this, gratitude inevitably leads us to becoming aware of the unlimited wealth that life holds for every one of us. Grateful people tend to be happier, more optimistic, more satisfied with their lives than their less grateful counterparts. Michael E. McCullough, a professor from Florida, provides experimental evidence that gratitude leads to improvements in psychological and even *physical* well-being.[1]

McCullough's groundbreaking research demonstrates that "people who place too much emphasis on materialistic pursuits—people for whom obtaining wealth and material possessions takes priority over meaningful relationships, community involvement, and spirituality—tend to be unhappy people. In general, they are dissatisfied with their lives, and tend to experience high levels of negative emotion. They are at risk for a variety of mental disorders. In contrast, grateful people—people who readily recognize the many ways in which their lives are enriched by the benevolent actions of others—tend to be extraordinarily happy. They experience high levels of positive emotion and are generally satisfied with their lives."[2]

Psychology demonstrates three main reasons that may lead people to higher materialistic pursuits:

1. **insecurity** that is formed when people don't have their basic psychological needs met, such as safety, competence, and connectedness.
2. **lack of confidence** formed from being raised in a family in which the parents were divorced or separated.
3. materialistic themes that flood modern society in the form of **advertisements,** compelling people to unconsciously assimilate money-oriented values. For example, television frequently presents unrealistic media images that reduce many viewers' life satisfaction.[3]

Being constantly exposed to a vast variety of advertising and financial challenges, we may increase our materialistic perception of life. According to McCullough's research, gratefulness is such a powerful approach to life that it may reduce people's materialistic strivings.[4]

I invite you to apply this valuable information about the power of gratitude to any situation in your life. Below, I present two different approaches to watching another person consume a cooked delicacy.

The materialistic approach:

What is that heavenly smell? Oh no! It's pizza! Look at how they are enjoying it. How come I am not allowed to enjoy it? Am I a monk? They don't look as if they are going to die. Can it be true that I will never again in my entire life be able to partake of such a pleasant meal? Oh, how lucky these fellows are! I wish I could enjoy pizza now as they do! What torture, poor me. Oh, that aroma ... it brings tears to my eyes. So many of the sweetest memories come to mind, the best times. Now they are over. E-eh.

The grateful approach:

That smell is oddly familiar. Wow, pizza. I had a lot of it in my life! More than one could dream of. Now it is time to take care of my health. Yeah, health is my priority now. All these people eating pizzas will be delighted to discover a healthy diet in their time. I am grateful that I am on a healthy diet already. I do feel a lot better. I am so glad that I will not have to be sick again. In only fifteen minutes I will be home. What do I have in my fridge? Those Hass avocados I bought yesterday should be perfectly ripe today. It will only take a couple of minutes to prepare guacamole with lemon, tomatoes, and jalapeño. Uh, my mouth is watering! I have fresh romaine lettuce, tomatoes, and a giant organic mango that will be so yummy and nourishing. Oh, I am looking forward to my raw dinner that will leave me feeling light and wonderful. I greatly appreciate what the raw-food diet is doing for my body and mind. How fortunate I am! What a blessing life is.

Practicing thankfulness is the most effective coping technique that I am aware of. To develop a grateful attitude, we need to practice one simple activity—notice the positive sides of events in our lives. The very best way to do this is to keep a gratitude journal. Buy yourself a notebook and start writing three to five grateful notes daily. I think that we should be grateful not only for the positive but also the negative experiences. Often it is the most painful events in our lives that shape the qualities in ourselves we value most. I met a person who kept his gratitude journal for ten years. He claimed that his life turned from misery to happiness, thanks to his journal. Other people keep their gratitude journals until they develop a subconscious, ongoing mental pattern of thankfulness. In one experiment, writing notes of appreciation led to increases in high-frequency heart rate variability in participants. The high-frequency band of the heart rate power spectrum is believed to reflect the input of the parasympathetic branch of the autonomic nervous system to the heart and is related to a variety of beneficial mental and physical health outcomes.[5]

The following exercise will help you to experience the powerful shift in how you feel from practicing gratitude:

Write or say three things that you are grateful for right now and carefully observe your feelings. Describe or write down your feelings.

Thankfulness goes side by side with forgiveness. Grateful people who are accustomed to seeing the brighter side of life are most likely to feel empathy towards the person who hurt them and be able to forgive the offender.

Research by the Gallup Organization found that 94% of Americans have prayed for forgiveness at some time.[6] Therefore, forgiveness appears to be important to nearly all of us. Like gratitude, fostering the quality of forgiveness is vital for experiencing a good life. Forgiveness requires giving up long-held resentments and negative judgments of transgressors, and sometimes it even requires the ability to be grateful for the hard lesson received. Forgiving transforms bitterness into a neutral feeling, or even a positive feeling, making it more feasible for us to feel happier.

In addition to having a positive impact on our happiness, forgiveness brings us better physical health. It may reduce depression and anxiety. Scientists recently discovered that when people ruminate about the offense they suffered, they experience a short-term increase in cortisol, which can result in mood swings, lack of motivation, loss of muscle, and loss of appetite.[7] Therefore, feelings of revenge or rumination can seriously undermine our ability to stay on a raw-food diet and consequently inhibit the healing process itself. On the other hand, practicing gratitude and forgiveness can make your life on a raw-food diet more enjoyable and will have a positive impact on your health, your mood, and your life in general.

ACTUALIZING DREAMS

"Dare to live the life you have dreamed for yourself."

—Ralph Waldo Emerson

Raw-fooders often say that raw food is not merely a diet but a lifestyle because it transforms most aspects of one's life. In addition to improving health, staying on a raw-food diet awards us with more time, more energy, and more money.

Time. Perhaps you will save the greatest amount of time by not getting sick and going to the doctor now and in the future. Furthermore, you will gain two to three hours per day from needing less sleep and no naps. The third big time saving will come from less cooking.

Ironically, most people believe that preparing raw food takes a long time. In my opinion, the only process that consumes time is learning to use the equipment: blender, processor, juicer, and dehydrator. The preparation process itself in most cases takes minutes. Raw cuisine totally excludes such time-consuming procedures as preheating the oven, baking, boiling, steaming, frying, sautéing, and of course washing and scrubbing greasy skillets, pots, pans, and the stove. Your sparkling clean stove is just sitting quietly in the corner of the kitchen, always cool and spotless, covered with jars of sprouts or a large cutting board. Washing the dishes after a raw-food meal also takes only minutes.

Some people are concerned that such procedures as dehydrating or sprouting are time-consuming. However, that is not the case. Despite the fact that it takes twenty-four hours or so for crackers to dry, we don't sit next to them waiting. To make the dough and lay out the crackers takes approximately half an hour, including clean-up. While the dehydrator runs, we can do whatever we want—go to work or have fun—the crackers will not burn. Growing sprouts works the same way: the sprouting process happens over two to three days, but putting seeds in the water and draining them about every twelve hours takes only one or two minutes.

Most raw-food preparation can be done in minutes. For example, to make a raw soup in a blender takes approximately sixty seconds, plus dicing and cleaning. If you have a powerful blender, it is not possible to blend anything non-stop for more than two minutes because the mixture in the blender will get too hot.

Of course, preparing raw food may take longer in the beginning, when you are first learning. You may not be an experienced peeler and chopper; the recipes may sound too confusing or complicated. Yet I would like to assure you that if you persist in practicing, you will quickly develop the skills of a raw chef: your recipes will become simple, you'll be able to use the equipment automatically (like driving), and in a matter of weeks you will become great at chopping and dicing.

You will also gain additional time from many other aspects of your "raw" life. For example, your shopping will take less time, as you make all of your purchases in one section now. You might need to buy fewer garments considering that your healthy body will look nice in almost any clothing. At work, when others take a snack break or a smoke break, you may choose to use this time for some valuable activity, such as a walk. On top of everything mentioned, you may move the entire aging process some years farther away. This probably adds another ten to fifteen years of lifetime, at your disposal.

Finally, you will notice that your mind becomes sharper, and you will make faster decisions. I have noticed that it takes me less time to fill out paperwork. I am able to concentrate better and thus perform any job more rapidly. Whether I am gardening, writing an article, cleaning my house, or working in my office, I can now work efficiently for many hours without needing a break. When I hire younger people who eat cooked food, I observe them getting tired too soon and needing breaks. I understand that due to consuming a healthy diet, even though I'm in my fifties, I possess more energy than some young people who consume a predominantly cooked-food diet.

Energy. Many years ago when I was eating cooked foods, I used to set my alarm clock to beep twice so I could wake up slowly, because no amount of sleep would make me feel fresh. Every time the clock beeped, I wanted to crush it. I would crawl out of bed an hour and a half prior to my appointments in the morning, because I needed to curl my hair, fix my face, dress up, put on perfume and deodorant, drink coffee, and I don't even remember what else. I only know that I never went for even a short walk. I looked sleepy and felt tired. Now, I can literally wake up fifteen minutes before I have to walk out the door, and I look fresh and feel energetic. Moreover, I never use the alarm clock anymore; I don't even have one! The sun fills the morning with light; I open my eyes and instantly wake up, usually long before any possible appointments; and I always have time to go for a walk.

Society is structured in such a way that people give the most productive part of their days to their jobs, which typically go from 9 a.m. to 5 p.m. Most people feel too tired after an eight-hour working day to do anything but watch TV, eat, and relax at home. By comparison, people who have been staying on the raw-food diet for as little as a couple of weeks testify that at the end of their work day, they feel as fresh as in the morning. Some of them continue to work vigorously for several more hours.

Before my family went on a raw-food diet, my husband Igor had three employees in his health spa. They were cleaning, raking leaves, mowing the grass, planting flowers, unloading wood from the truck and chopping it for the sauna, vacuuming the rooms, laundering, folding towels, and making refreshments for the customers. After only two months on a raw-food diet, Igor took over the entire load of work himself because he now has enough energy to perform these jobs alone.

On Igor's forty-ninth birthday, he was presented with two bars on which to do push-ups. At first he was not very excited. He told us how he used to dream of doing a hundred push-ups at one time when he was sixteen years old, because he wanted to impress a pretty girl. Despite practicing diligently and consuming lots of protein, young Igor could only achieve seventy push-ups in one trial. After such an intense workout, his arms were left shaking and aching. That was why Igor gave up and didn't even try to do push-ups for more than thirty years. Now he was wondering how many push-ups he could do on these bars. He was guessing maybe ten or twenty. The next morning Igor decided to check it out. He did fifty push-ups right away, stood up, and went around the push-up bars. Then he did fifty more, and more, and more. I came in after three hours to tell him that we needed to go. Igor was still doing push-ups and got upset with me, because he had almost made a thousand!

Since that time, Igor has been carrying his push-up bars with him everywhere. He does push-ups at the gas station while pumping the gas, and at the parking lot while waiting for me to do the shopping. He is still trying to figure out what his highest score could be. When he gets bored with push-ups, he jumps-rope into the hundreds. I am sure that when Olympic athletes discover the raw-food diet, many of the world records might be impressively broken.

Money. Before my family went on a raw-food diet, we spent hundreds and sometimes thousands of dollars every month on bills from doctors and dentists, for medicine and medical devices, and for health insurance. We must also consider the money we lost from the days we missed work being sick. If I were to take the lowest number and multiply it for all the years we have been on a healthy diet, the amount would come to many thousands of dollars. All these years we have not had any medical insurance. Hence, we can afford organic papayas and pineapples.

In addition to these major savings, you may save additional funds by simplifying your lifestyle. For example, after several months of staying on a raw-food diet, you may begin to eat simpler and spend less money on your meals. You may choose to turn your heaters off and sleep with an open window. You may decide to use fewer chemicals in your household, along with eliminating most air fresheners, deodorants, and cosmetics.

We have already discussed how people may gain more time and energy by adopting a raw-food diet. If desired, you may transfer these savings into further monetary income.

As you may see, additional time, energy, and money arrive as an extra bonus of becoming a raw-foodist. In comparison, I recall that when I ate a diet of predominantly cooked foods, I had a constant deficit of time, energy, and money. I was stuck in a vicious circle: lacking money, I needed to work more; as a result I didn't have time or energy left for creative, playful activities. Being emotionally drained from such a boring life, I was too tired to do anything creative, and so I ate more often. To pay for stimulating foods, I had to again work more, and so on. I felt exhausted and unsatisfied.

Adopting a raw-food lifestyle turned out to be a multi-dimensional present for everyone in my family. I am aware of many people whose lives have been dramatically enhanced on various levels by switching to a raw-food diet. For example, my friend Rhonda, mother of four, used to be a real estate agent. After becoming a raw-foodist, she studied to be a midwife, first as a hobby and later as a main job. Now Rhonda educates pregnant women about eating well and helps mothers give birth to healthy babies. She claims that adopting a raw-food diet started a new, more meaningful chapter in her life.

I believe that by going on a raw-food diet, every person receives a unique opportunity to actualize his or her most sacred dreams. This Step—Actualizing Dreams—is about getting prepared for a big move towards a more fulfilling life. I believe it is important to plan how you are going to spend your bonus time, energy, and money. As paradoxical as it sounds, having extra time could be a problem. Participants in my workshops often tell me that they don't know what to do with extra time. Being bored, they keep checking the fridge because food continually comes into their mind. However, one cannot eat two buckets of almonds the way one used to consume popcorn, nor can one eat as many raisins as M&Ms. Raw food is so much richer in nutrients, the body feels full more quickly. As a result, people cannot entertain themselves with food as they used to. They begin to feel deprived of the fun of snacking and soon get off the raw-food diet. Finding other pleasurable activities seems to be the only working alternative to this puzzle.

Here is another typical story. When Jennifer started having more free time, she found it difficult not to think about eating. She described how she would wake up early in the morning full of energy, walk the dog, pace around the house looking for things to do, cut a bush in the garden, start laundry, jump on the rebounder, watch a little TV, then look at the clock and find that it was only 8:30 a.m. At this point Jennifer became frustrated and puzzled because she couldn't think of anything else to do.

Meanwhile, many people tell me that they have had certain dreams for as long as they can remember but they never had the chance to follow their visions, because they didn't have enough time, energy, and money.

If you don't know which activity to choose, pay attention to what other people create out of inspiration. Most importantly, try choosing activities that are useful for your community and Earth-friendly. Go to your local YMCA, community college, or recreational center for ideas and see what attracts your heart. Please find below some activities that people from my workshops have listed as their dreams.

- To plant many fruit trees in town
- To write a book

- To teach neighborhood children to read
- To cater raw food
- To take care of animals
- To learn how to construct cob houses
- To do art work
- To learn sign language
- To get involved in a community theater production
- To make raw crackers for sale
- To go on a long hike with a friend
- To plant an organic garden
- To sew dolls and send them to children in poor countries
- To volunteer in church
- To bike across the state as a fundraiser for a good cause
- To take voice lessons and to sing at community events
- To study the geology in one's region
- To sing in a choir

Staying on a raw-food diet may enrich us in many ways. In addition to better health, we can gain more time, energy, and money. You may use these riches in any way you like. Your choice may influence your life and can make a difference in the whole world. May all your dreams come true!

EMBRACING OTHER HEALTHY HABITS

"Sickness is the vengeance of nature for the violation of her laws."

—Charles Simmons

While diet is a key factor in human health, there are many more important aspects to optimal health. I consider the following components to be the most vital for human well-being:

- Exercise
- Sunshine
- Good sleep
- Proper breathing
- Drinking pure water
- Stress management
- Tempering the body with cold water

Exercise. Medical researchers at Harvard and Stanford universities, after studying the habits and health of 17,000 middle-aged and older men, reported the first scientific evidence that even modest exercise helps prolong life.[1]

If one generation is twenty years, then there have been only five hundred generations since 10,000 BC. Therefore, we inherited our current genetic design from our ancestors who lived thousands of years ago. If we aren't living a physically active lifestyle, our bodies may react in a negative way. When we sit around and live sedentary, inactive lifestyles, our bodies weaken and we can become seriously ill even if we eat healthy. Therefore if you can dedicate at least thirty minutes of your day to performing exercise or some form of physically intensive work, you will receive some or all of the following benefits:

• Increased energy
• Improved metabolism
• An increase in muscles
• Reduced stress
• Improved self-esteem
• Less body fat
• The reduced risk of many serious diseases, such as cancer, heart disease, arthritis, diabetes, and osteoporosis
• An increase in blood circulation

Sunshine. For centuries, doctors and natural healers relied on medical treatment by sunlight (called "heliotherapy") to help heal many common ailments. Scientific research shows sunshine to be an effective treatment for rickets, osteomalacia, osteoporosis, acne, eczema, psoriasis, neonatal jaundice, and depression. Without the sun's life-giving energy we are at thirty times greater risk of death from cancer.[2]

I came upon an article in a medical journal that discussed the benefits of adequate sunlight. In an experiment with twelve hundred children who were exposed to various levels of sunlight, exposure to adequate amounts of sunshine led to an 80% reduction in developing diabetes in comparison with the control group.

This article explained that vitamin D from fish cannot substitute for sunshine.[3]

According to an article in the *Washington Post*, "Many Americans, particularly African Americans, may be suffering from unrecognized deficiencies of a key nutrient—vitamin D—that increase the risk of bone problems and a host of other diseases. Some evidence suggests that a lack of vitamin D may be associated with many forms of cancer, high blood pressure, depression, and immune-system disorders such as multiple sclerosis, rheumatoid arthritis, and diabetes."[4]

We need to be exposed to sunlight regularly because it heals and supports one's body in the following beneficial ways:

- Lowered cholesterol
- Lowered blood pressure
- Improved thyroid functioning
- Regulated immune system
- Improved insulin production
- Improved heart muscle contractility

I recommend to everyone the regular, preferably daily, practice of sunbathing for at least thirty to sixty minutes, especially for those people who work indoors under artificial lighting. However, I would like to warn against exposure to extreme sunshine, such as in the middle of the day in the summer, particularly in regions located close to the equator or at high altitudes.

Good Sleep. Human beings were created in a very smart and prophetic way. Our Creator predicted that we humans would engage in different kinds of abuse and do harm to our health during the active part of our days. Therefore, our Creator magically blessed us with the need for sleep every night so that no matter what we do in the daytime, during the dark hours sleep prevents us from continuing the insanity of the day. Every single person in the world must lie down and stay motionless for several hours each night. We are unable to drink, smoke, or overeat when we are asleep. No matter what damage we do to ourselves in the daytime, at night our bodies heal themselves.

Our bodies are trying to reach homeostasis during the night hours in order to heal. However, we humans have succeeded in our destructive behavior during the day to such a degree that it even impairs our nighttime sleep. Very often we don't realize how little things can harm our health. I would like to share several recommendations with you.

1. Whenever possible, sleep in the fresh air: fresh outside air is rich in negative ions. Elevated negative air-ion levels are widely reported to have beneficial effects on humans, including enhanced feelings of relaxation and reduced levels of tiredness, stress, irritability, depression, and tenseness.[5] My entire family and I try to sleep outside year-round. My husband built a structure in our back yard, a combination of a gazebo and a shed that has big windows without glass, a huge open door, and even an opening just beneath the roof. That is where my family sleeps when we are at home. Whenever it's not raining, we don't even sleep in this structure—we sleep outside on the deck directly under the stars.

2. Let your energy field restore. Our energy field expands several feet beyond our body in the shape of a gigantic egg. This energy field is our cradle of healing. At night any damage is repaired, but not if we have an alarm clock next to our head, or computers

running in our bedroom. All electrical devices have an electromagnetic field that extends out for several feet beyond their physical structure. When the two fields cross, the body cannot fully heal. I personally turn off all electrical fixtures if I have to sleep indoors. I'm also careful about refrigerators, microwaves, or other strong devices running in an adjacent room because the plywood wall does not stop those harmful vibrations.

3. Sleep on a hard surface: our bodies need to stretch out at night. All the bones and joints can only stretch out when we lie on a hard surface. This is especially important for the spine. During the day, the spine is improperly positioned while driving, sitting in front of the computer, and watching TV, such that some spinal joints don't get adequate spinal fluid and blood enriched with oxygen. My entire family prefers to sleep on hard beds or on the floor in sleeping bags. You should see us sleeping on the floor around the king-sized bed in hotels when we travel. If we are forced by circumstances to sleep on soft beds, we wake up with headaches, feeling achy, and not rested.

4. Don't go to sleep on a full stomach. Try to eat your last meal at least two to three hours before you go to bed and aim to eat light food so that it is digested by the time you fall asleep.

5. Learn to sleep in the nude: any clothing, no matter how loose, interferes with the circulation of blood while you sleep. Synthetic nightwear is especially harmful because it accumulates static electricity, which interferes with the body's energy.

6. Sleep at night: no wonder the night shifts in the U.S. are called the "graveyard shifts." It is very important to sleep at night. The human body is attuned to the movement of the stars and the universe, and different organs rest at different hours of the day. For

example, the adrenal glands rest best between 11 p.m. and 1 a.m. That is when we begin to feel so sleepy that we use coffee, loud music, and bright lights to stay awake. If we try to stay up after 11 p.m. as a habit, our adrenals eventually wear out and as a result, we could feel sleepy and tired during the day. Over the years of habitual staying awake late, one might develop insomnia and depression.

I understand that we all lead busy lives and these little things might seem unimportant. I recommend that you try improving your sleeping conditions and see how the quality of your sleep will improve from following these simple guidelines. I work very hard and some days feel exhausted when I go to bed. I take care of my sleep and wake up refreshed, full of energy, and in a good mood.

Proper Breathing. Oxygen plays a vital role in the circulatory and respiratory systems. As we breathe, oxygen that is inhaled nourishes the body and purifies the blood by removing poisonous waste products circulating throughout our blood system. According to Michael White, founder of The Optimal Breathing Development System,* "the respiratory system is responsible for eliminating 70% of our metabolic waste." Irregular breathing may hinder this purification process and cause waste products to remain in circulation, which may contribute to many serious illnesses.

Based on years of research, White states: "Most people have unhealthy breathing habits. They hold their breath or breathe high in the chest or in a shallow, irregular manner. These patterns have been unconsciously adopted, accidentally formed, or emotionally

---

*Michael White's educational website: www.breathing.com

impressed. Certain 'typical' breathing patterns may trigger physiological and psychological stress and anxiety reactions."[6]

To check your own pattern of breathing, sit in a quiet place and relax for a minute or two. Put your hand, horizontally, about one inch above your navel. Close your eyes. Breathe normally without trying to influence your breathing one way or the other. Observe how your abdomen moves every time you breathe in and out. If you are breathing correctly, you should find that the hand over the stomach moves as you breathe in and out.

Abdominal breathing is the correct way of breathing. If your chest is moving as you breathe, and you do not have a medical reason to do so, that means that you are breathing shallowly and incorrectly.

Begin paying steady attention to your breathing. Any time you find yourself holding your breath, breathing irregularly or too rapidly, go back to your abdominal breathing.

Drinking Pure Water. Presence of an adequate amount of water in the human body ensures that every system of the body functions normally. Water makes up more than two-thirds of the weight of the human body. Without it, humans die in a few days. Water makes up 95% of the human brain, 82% of our blood, and 90% of our lungs. As a result of extensive research into the role of water in the body, Dr. Fereydoon Batmanghelidj has found chronic dehydration to be the cause of many conditions including asthma, allergies, arthritis, angina, migraine headaches, hypertension, raised cholesterol, chronic fatigue syndrome, multiple sclerosis, depression, false hunger, and diabetes in the elderly.[7] The main health benefits of water include:

- More energy
- Better metabolism

- A reduction in headaches and dizziness
- The loss of extra weight
- More efficient digestion and conversion of food into energy
- Better elimination of waste
- The lubrication of joints
- Better regulation of the body's temperature

Considering the fact that water content in a raw-food diet is relatively high, you do not need to drink eight glasses of water per day, unless you consume a lot of salt, live in a dry climate, and/or exercise heavily for prolonged periods of time. I usually drink about four glasses of water a day. Sometimes, when I consume two or three quarts of green smoothie in a day, I drink very little or no water at all. Of course, you need to choose only the best pure water for your consumption.

Stress Management. When we worry or experience stress, our bodies turn on the same physiological responses that animal bodies do, but we do not resolve conflict in the same way—through fighting or fleeing. Over time, the constant activation of a stress response makes us literally sick. In his best-selling book, *Why Zebras Don't Get Ulcers*, Dr. Robert Sapolsky explains how prolonged stress causes or intensifies a range of physical and mental afflictions, including depression, ulcers, colitis, heart disease, and more.[8]

As I mentioned above, I consider walking to be an effective natural way of handling stress. If you don't like walking, you may practice other forms of exercise. I prefer walking because it is the most natural movement for all humans, and it is good both for the mind and the body. Walking relieves stress because it provides a way for the body to release tension and built-up frustration by raising the output of endorphins—one of the "feel good" chemicals in the brain.

Many stresses can be changed, eliminated, or minimized. Here are some things you can do to reduce your level of stress:

- Become aware of your own reactions to stress.
- Reinforce positive self-statements.
- Focus on your good qualities and accomplishments.
- Avoid unnecessary competition.
- Develop assertive behaviors.
- Recognize and accept your limits. Remember that everyone is unique and different.
- Talk with friends or someone you can trust about your worries/ problems.
- Learn to use your time wisely.
- Practice relaxation techniques. For example, whenever you feel tense, slowly breathing in and out for several minutes may help you to relax.[9]

Tempering the Body with Cold Water. Throughout history, humans bathed exclusively in cold water except on those rare occasions when they had access to hot springs. Today there are still many places where people have only cold water for their personal use.

Ancient Greeks were aware of the healing properties of cold water. When they invented the first water-heating systems in 700 BC, they continued using cold-water treatments for health purposes. Spartans, for whom health was a matter of high reputation, considered it unmanly to use hot water; they regularly dipped in cold water for vigor and better health.[10]

In the first century AD, in Finland it became common for people to jump into cold streams or lakes after sweating in saunas. The indigenous peoples of ancient Russia used cold plunges into icy water for the ceremony of "purification" in the ninth century. Tempering the body with cold water has been a widespread Russian tradition throughout the centuries and into the present.[11]

Swimming in ice water is such a large part of Russian culture and tradition that there is even a major government-funded organization called The Federation of Tempering and Winter Swimming. In addition, Moscow hosts an annual science conference dedicated to researching the influence of cold water on the human organism. There are several research institutes in Russia, especially in Siberia, that have been studying the effects of cold temperatures on human health for many decades. I would like to share some of their findings.

The maximum healing occurs when the body is submerged in water with a temperature *below* 12° Celsius (53° F) for one to two minutes.[12] During the brief application of cold water, the blood vessels in the skin abruptly contract, pushing a large amount of blood inside the organism. This results in the re-activating of the inner capillaries, many of which are typically atrophied by the age of thirty, due to poor circulation and an unhealthy lifestyle. The regeneration of a large amount of capillaries ensures that our inner organs receive the necessary nutrients for their optimal performance and rejuvenation. This great improvement in capillary circulation results in the younger appearance of cold-water swimmers.[13] In ancient Greece this process was called "the natural gymnastics of blood vessels."

Several scientific studies have demonstrated that within fifty seconds after the brief application of extremely cold temperatures, an enormous amount of heat is generated by the transformation of neurons, which is known as the phenomenon of "instant free heat."

Therefore, despite the initial shock that can be painful, winter swimmers (often called "Polar Bears") almost immediately experience an amazingly pleasant warmth from head to toe, causing the profound relaxation of the entire body.[14] This relaxation is one of a kind, as it cannot be compared to any other way of relaxing.

Russian scientists have demonstrated that the combination of quick cold stress and the resulting heat stimulates the body to find diseased cells and destroy them, thus reversing many degenerative diseases of liver, kidneys, and heart, as well as mental problems.[15]

After a cold plunge, the surface of the skin becomes charged with negative ions. Russian academician and scientist Alexander Chizhevsky considered this charge of negative ions to be important for our bodies, which are often charged too positively.[16]

Tempering the body with cold water increases the rate of the metabolism. This brings about the purging of free radicals, heavy metals, nitrates, and pesticides. Additionally, this cleansing occurs via skin and lungs, thereby unloading the burden on the kidneys.[17]

Finally, swimming in cold water dramatically strengthens immunity. While constantly protecting ourselves from natural cold and heat by using air conditioners, heaters, and clothing, we keep our bodies at the same temperature, disabling our natural system of thermal regulation. We tend to think that this brings our body to a healthy and comfortable state when in actuality, the opposite is true. When exposed to cold temperatures, a human organism that has not been trained to regulate its internal temperature loses its internal heat approximately thirty times faster than a tempered body.[18] As a result, one can get sick from even minor changes in outside temperatures—for example, after waiting five extra minutes in windy weather or after getting wet in the rain.

Meanwhile, we have not even remotely explored the depth of human abilities. My mind was totally blown away when I read a report of the new sport named "Aquaice": swimming in ice-cold water, which became popular in recent years in Russia, Japan, Czech Republic, China, and other countries. Hundreds of competitors take part in marathon swims in ice-cold water, usually lasting for many hours. For example, as soon as the thick ice cracked on the Moscow River on March 19, 2006, twenty teams from different regions of Russia competed in a 100-kilometer (62.1-mile) swim. The teams consisted of four swimmers (men and women) who took turns covering this distance. The record time was 42 hours, 45 minutes! The longest stretch was 7,000 meters (4.3 miles). In order to reach this level of tempering in the body it takes several years of constant practice.[19]

Cold-water swimming is becoming increasingly popular in many places, including North America. There is a number of old Polar Bear Clubs in the state of New York that engage hundreds of people in this healthy practice.

Perhaps the biggest Polar Bear Club on this continent is located in Vancouver, BC, where thousands of people are involved. For instance, on New Year's Day in the year 2000, there were 2,128 "Polar Bears" simultaneously swimming in the ice-cold ocean to celebrate.[20]

In the 1980s, my husband Igor was president of the regional Polar Bear Club in Moscow. He took our family every morning before work to swim in frozen rivers and lakes, including the times I was pregnant and breastfeeding. I remember how we got so used to our cold baths that we couldn't miss even one day. If we skipped dipping in the ice water for one day there was a definite feeling of loss, and the children didn't sleep well and exhibited cranky behavior. I personally felt that the whole day went wrong.

Winter swimming is a wonderful method of tempering the body, which increases the energetic strength of the organism. Statistics hold that among those who practice winter swimming, sickness rates decrease for cold-type diseases by *sixty times*.[21] As a therapeutic method, winter swimming can heal many illnesses, including arthritis, hypertension, tuberculosis, type 2 diabetes, chronic gastrointestinal diseases, different inflammations, menstrual cycle abnormalities, dermatitis, and many others. Of course, everyone should receive proper instructions at the local Polar Bear Club or from the literature before jumping in a cold river.

Some researchers question the benefits of human exposure to very cold and hot temperatures as too extreme. I believe that these practices are as natural for people as exercising or fasting. For example, feeling tired after jogging doesn't mean that we should abstain from running. Both the facts and research show that people who try to always stay in the same temperature range by using heaters, air conditioning, or warm clothes often end up having less energy, vitality, and longevity.[22] Most centenarians (people one hundred years old and above) live in the mountains where the contrast of temperature is unavoidable.

Contrary to popular belief, winter swimming is remarkably enjoyable. After dipping in cold water I feel so good and refreshed that I cannot think of anything else being compatible with this pleasure. My family traditionally goes for a swim on each New Year's morning. Igor has introduced dozens of Americans to cold-water swimming. Many participants of our retreats in Ashland experienced jumping into the cold river and told us that they felt incredibly energized and pleased with the whole experience.

Step 10

GAINING CLARITY

"Clarity of mind means clarity of passion, too; this is why a great and clear mind loves ardently and sees distinctly what it loves."

—Blaise Pascal

I consider clarity to be the biggest gift we can have. When I say "clarity," I don't mean "the ability to understand the meanings of words and scientific definitions," or "to have a vast speaking vocabulary." To me, "clarity" is "the ability to see things as they are, to be able to separate truth from deception on my own, to know what I want and what I need."

Following a raw-food diet has helped me discover clarity. Since I began eating raw foods, I stopped being a typical member of society because most people in the world believe that eating cooked food is healthy. My habits and behaviors have been continuously changing. My lifestyle differs from the way the majority of people live. Often I am compelled to make serious decisions on my own. In the beginning, the constant need to decide by myself was new, and even scary. Periodically I panicked and searched for ready answers from "experts." But there are no true experts in the "raw-food world." We are all pioneers. Gradually I discovered that making my own decisions was not as dangerous and doomed to failure as I expected. On the contrary, deciding for myself appeared to be safer, more enjoyable, and led to more fruitful results.

My whole perception of life began shifting. Many of my favorite beliefs began to seem false. Some of my opinions stopped making sense, and in place of my former knowledge, *clarity* came. For example, I used to believe that everyone should always finish the food on their plate, because children in China and Africa are starving to death. Suddenly it occurred to me that forcing myself to overeat doesn't make any difference to those poor children. Another of my seemingly solid opinions was that I have to please everyone else before I can please myself. One day I had a revelation that to keep myself happy was one of the main missions in my life.

Now it is hard for me to imagine how I was able to live without clarity until I was thirty-eight years old. I was convinced that I was incapable of creating a new thought or coming up with a new conclusion completely on my own. I was sure that I could only read or hear clever ideas from other very smart people. I tried to accumulate knowledge, collecting many professional points of view, memorizing facts and quotes. I composed my lectures and articles from other people's lectures and books. My idea of "wisdom" and "intelligence" was "to possess as many pieces of information in my mind as possible." I believed the cliché: "Knowledge is power." At the same time, I could not understand why no matter how hard I tried, my lectures were not popular and my articles were boring even to me. Discouraged, I lost interest and stopped teaching and writing for many years.

When I began experiencing glimpses of clarity, and I was moved to share some of my own discoveries, I was amazed by the attention I received from other people that I had never before experienced. With glowing eyes, my listeners were asking for more. People in my audience and I experienced profound inspiration, and I fell in love with lecturing. I am thankful that I can clearly see that *knowledge can never substitute for clarity.* Knowledge is not even information. Knowledge is someone's opinion. Clarity is the ability to see life events as they are, without the distortion of knowledge. Very often, accumulated knowledge prevents us from gaining real clarity. I am glad that I have a lot of clarity now. In my life, I do not have to depend on experts or authorities to make my decisions. I know what I need to eat and drink, how I need to sleep, and what to wear, what to read. And I know the answer to the most important question of all: "What do I want to do in my life?"

I don't think we can benefit from other people seeing and thinking for us, but sometimes we can be inspired by their ideas. For example, Einstein told the world: "Everything is relative." When I consider his idea, I can see clearly that my own viewpoint is the only vision of reality I can trust.

Very often we confuse *clarity* with "ostentatious words." I would like to explain. If I, for example, memorized an entire textbook on human anatomy and even if I could retell anything from that book, it still doesn't mean that I have *clarity* about how the human body functions. Most of us have lots of knowledge and very little *clarity.* When we don't understand the difference between the two, we prefer to have knowledge rather than clarity. Clarity starts when we pay close attention to the intricate shifts of our feelings and impressions while observing the objective experience without hiding behind pleasant illusions. Clarity enables us to deal with the root of each situation in the most optimal way.

With clarity, we can see the spiritual nature of human beings. With clarity, we can feel oneness with all living things. With clarity, we can feel true happiness. When we are truly happy, we don't look for pleasures. Only unhappy people are focused on pleasures. Happiness is a part of the natural law.

To gain clarity, you may practice *de-conditioning*. Throughout our lives, we have all accumulated conditioning that obscures clarity. "To be conditioned" means "to have firm opinions that were formed in the past." "To de-condition oneself" means "to form fresh images of subjects or ideas every time we encounter them." In other words, "to be unconditioned" means "to live in the present." For example, when we began living next to the mountain, at first we admired the beautiful view every minute we noticed it. After some time, we stopped seeing that mountain. We become conditioned to know that it was there. Guests notice the mountain because they have a fresh, unconditioned approach to it. They tell us, "You live in such a gorgeous place!" We can start noticing the mountain again if we look at it every day with fresh eyes.

In order to de-condition ourselves, we need to be able to see as many conditionings in ourselves as possible. This sharing from my workshop might give you ideas of different conditioning:

- I used to be conditioned to think that animals don't feel pain.
- I used to be conditioned that failure is bad.
- I used to be ashamed of being poor.
- I used to be ashamed that my parents were very wealthy.
- I used to be conditioned to think that men are smarter than women.
- I used to be conditioned to think that I had to drink milk every day to have calcium.
- I used to be conditioned to think that I have to answer the phone each time it rings.
- I was conditioned to believe that I had to eat a lot to grow big.

- I used to be conditioned to think that I must have a career to be successful.
- I used to be conditioned to think that a woman's place was in the kitchen.
- I used to be conditioned to think that it was my teacher's *job* to make me smart.
- I used to be conditioned to think that money would make me happy.
- I used to be conditioned to think that children should be seen and not heard.
- I used to believe that good grades were the priority of my education.
- I used to be conditioned to think that I have to drink to be social.
- I used to be conditioned to think that when other people were sad they lacked my advice.

When we begin questioning our beliefs, we may discover thousands of thoughts that no longer reflect our present perception of life. Then we may clearly see how this conditioning has been shaping our life, adding helplessness and frustration to it. The good thing is that we do not have to fight our conditioning but only to see it clearly. The minute we observe an erroneous thought, it disappears and the clarity comes into place. Clarity is our precious ability to observe reality as it is, without any distortion.

SEARCHING FOR ONE'S SPIRITUAL MISSION

"There is more hunger for love and appreciation in this world than for bread."

—Mother Teresa

We are all spiritual beings. I know this because I feel a spiritual connection every time I look into another person's eyes. Not only do we feel this unexplainable and immeasurable energy from humans, we can also feel these same deep vibrations from animals and plants. For example, have you seen how a blade of grass makes its way through a thick layer of dirt, clay, and rock? It's difficult to believe that such a tender plant could overcome seemingly solid ground. I cannot find any explanation for this phenomenon other than the invisible yet powerful energy that comes from the sprout in an effort to survive in spite of obstruction.

All living things are connected, and we communicate using different energies and vibrations. Think about Canadian geese, which are able to fly long distances and find certain lakes without ever being mistaken. I am fascinated by their powerful ability to navigate without compasses or other tools, using their incredible instincts. Another example comes from my encounters with dogs. Instinctively, they always know when I am afraid of them. They are also able to transmit their mood to me, so I may recognize that they are totally aware of my emotions. Several times I have had powerful experiences with cats. I consider them small and fairly safe animals to approach, but once in a while, before I even decide to reach out with my hand and pet a cat, it sends a ray of energy that warns me to back off—without even curling its back or hissing. I bring up these examples to illustrate that every one of us, all the time, deals with energies that are not visible but nevertheless very powerful.

Why are we given these vast energies? I believe that these powers are given to us for a great purpose or mission. I believe that all human beings have their own mission in life. I also believe that to fulfill that mission is the most important purpose for every person because only then can one contribute the *most* to the rest of humanity. People who are able to do so mark history as the most gifted leaders in their profession.

How do we determine what our mission is? I think we can guess by observing our personal gifts and talents. Every single person has some particular talent. I have been working as an employer or director of various companies for more than twenty years, and I have noticed that all my employees have one gift or another. I've worked with dozens of people and have never met even one without talents. Usually, when I get to know people more closely, I find that they have more gifts than I expected. We definitely have different gifts and different missions in life.

For example, my husband loves to give massages. He always carries several massage tables in his truck. Igor doesn't care if he gets paid. Massage is his passion. Every day, he is looking for someone to rub. If Igor and I work on a project together, he offers me a massage several times a day. If I agree to it, he will massage me until I ask him to stop, and then he will feel sorry that it is over. Igor can talk for hours about how he loves to touch people and feel their energy. It is interesting that he cannot massage just anyone, but only certain people with whom he feels a connection. That is why Igor is not giving massages for a living. His massage sessions with people are so incredible that my husband is surrounded by legends wherever he goes. Sometimes after Igor gives me a massage, I make a feeble attempt to give a massage back to him, but my massages usually fail. One time, I honestly tried hard to learn massage, living next to such a great master, but I don't have enough strength and I get tired and bored in the first few minutes. As much as I appreciate him, I myself don't like to give massages at all. I wouldn't give massages even for a lot of money.

My passion is participating in sincere conversations with other people. When I listen to another human being, I forget about time, food, and sleep. Igor praises my patience with people, which I don't even notice. For all the money in the world, he says, he could not "listen to the same stuff over and over for hours." We have lived together for many years, we have a lot in common, and yet each one of us continues to carry on with our own passions through life.

Luckily, both my husband and I have found a way to make a living that lets us utilize our passions. It took us many years to realize that doing what we love is more important to us than the amount of money we could make. We had to learn to live on less money, but the joy we get from doing what we love means far more to us than money.

Often I read different reports in newspapers about people who don't like their job. They are suffering, counting the hours and minutes until lunch, a break, or the end of the working day. They are spending their lives waiting, waiting for the *end*. Why can't we do what we love? Why can't we live more enjoyable lives? I find two main answers to these questions:

1. People don't know what they love to do.
2. People consider their life passions to be unimportant.

In either case, people often do something they don't like, hoping to get back to their passion upon retiring. Or they do what they love, but they apply their talents to destructive processes instead of creative ones. For example, I have a friend who is a very good salesman. He claims that he could sell ice to an Eskimo. Obviously he is very talented if he can inspire people to buy things they don't need. I think that his real talent is to inspire people. I told him that he would make a great teacher or motivational leader, that he could inspire people to do beautiful, creative deeds. When he heard these words, he cried and told me that it was his secret dream to be a teacher, but he was afraid of poverty. Another friend of mine is a gifted artist. Her paintings are unique and beautiful and they touch the heart. However, she has not created a new painting for many years, because she can make more money designing for commercial and promotional advertising.

When I observe people participating in destructive businesses and activities, manufacturing environmentally harmful products, pouring chemicals into fields, distributing cotton candy in amusement parks, shooting B movies, and many more thoughtless and harmful actions, it becomes clear to me that these people don't understand the huge importance of following their mission. If a single blade of grass has the power to grow through the ground, one can only imagine the potential power of human energy applied with passion.

How many people can you name who have made a significant positive difference for the whole world? For example: Martin Luther King, Jr., Mahatma Gandhi, Byron Katie, Jiddu Krishnamurti, Leo Tolstoi, Mother Teresa, Eckhart Tolle, Paul McCartney, etc. These people passionately followed their life's mission. I believe that anybody could start following his or her life mission at any time and make a wonderful difference in the world.

Because we are spiritual beings, our spiritual missions are more important for our spirit than obtaining money for other than spiritual needs. When we do not follow our true goals, we develop spiritual pain, which we feel as boredom and emptiness. Since as early as childhood, many of us begin to feel bored once in a while. It often happens when we are forced to do things that we don't like, or when we are unable to do what we are passionate about. There is a vast difference between pleasurable activities such as watching television and visiting amusement parks, and things that help us evolve spiritually such as creatively working on projects that one has talents for. After watching movies, we often feel drained and even more bored, while after working creatively, we feel empowered, inspired, and fulfilled. We try to find the means that will give us a break from feeling senseless and empty. With years of disconnection from our life mission, our spiritual pains accumulate. Sometimes we have attacks of feeling lost, lonely, bored with life, or losing sense in life. Often this pain is blamed on life problems such as loneliness, troublesome relationships, debt, disease, etc. Spiritual pain can be worse than physical pain and can become unbearable. Most suicides happen because of spiritual pain, not physical pain. In America alone twenty-eight million people are taking antidepressants to be able to live through the day.[1] Yet it is everyone's birthright to be happy.

I invite you to observe the feelings you encounter while performing various tasks, and let your passions guide your life. For example, can you remember if you ever had a situation when you were enjoying doing something to such an extent that you completely forgot about time, missed lunch, and didn't care what other people thought of you? That was probably something that can give you an idea of what you should be doing more in your life. The spiritual awakening runs like a thread through all existing 12-Step programs. Staying away from cooked food is no exception. If you quit eating cooked food but keep suffering from loneliness and boredom, you will have lost your escape from spiritual pain and, being unable to face the emptiness, you might simply find another addiction to take the place of the former one such as shopping, gambling, watching TV, overworking, etc. That is why I have dedicated several steps in this program to spiritual awakening.

GIVING SUPPORT TO OTHERS

"There is no better way to thank God for your sight than by giving a helping hand to someone in the dark."

—Helen Keller

We rarely remember our first encounter with a raw-food diet, when one of our friends confided about his or her special lifestyle. Perhaps this person inspired us enough to sign up for the lecture of a famous raw-food teacher or loaned us a book written by a renowned raw-fooder. Later, it never occurs to us to whom we should be grateful to in the first place. Please take a moment to remember the first person in your life who told you about raw food. Send this person your gratitude. Without this person, you would never have gone to that lecture or read that first book. My first personal encounter with raw food happened in line at my bank, with Elizabeth, whose last name I don't even know. I would like to specially thank all the "first persons" who do the grassroots work in the world without being mentioned or rewarded or paid. I praise these people for their empathy with other people. Over and over again, they keep patiently answering all the same questions: "Where do you get your protein?" and "So you eat raw meat?" and "Don't you ever miss pizza?" I make my living by writing books and teaching classes about raw food, and I know that I wouldn't even have an audience without the heart-warming network that these enthusiasts have created.

Now *you* have the chance to contribute your support. It is your turn to be patient and empathetic towards other people. Let me clarify that I don't encourage you to jump on everyone in the street with the radical concepts of raw food. By the words "giving support" I do not mean making major repairs for someone, but rather "planting seeds in fertile soil"—helping those who are already seeking the natural lifestyle. Often after attending a lecture on the benefits of a raw-food diet, people try to convert desperately ill people, especially cancer patients, to this diet. They call me on the phone and request, "You need to talk to this person. She has cancer!" They assume that dangerously ill people are all ready for a change. My personal observation proves that the opposite is true. If people haven't started making healthy changes before they get seriously ill, they are unlikely to make changes while they are being closely watched by doctors. I recommend assisting people who are already willing to change their lifestyle.

There is no better way to introduce people to the idea of a raw-food diet (to plant a seed) than to feed them delicious raw food. Remember the very first raw meal that impressed you. Do you remember how you were thinking that maybe you could really eat this way? Was this experience important to you? Good-tasting raw food seems to be a turning point in most people's lives. The way to the heart may, after all, be through the stomach.

Giving support to others—this Step is about helping yourself while supporting others. This Step will support you in several ways. First of all, you strongly validate and greatly reinforce your own lifestyle by sharing it with friends. Second, it is always best to learn by teaching others. Finally, having more raw-fooders on our planet will make a world of difference, not only for them but for you as well. For example, how would you like to be able to dine out in a raw-food restaurant everywhere you go? Select a raw meal while flying in an airplane? Give a dollar to your child for a raw lunch at school? View billboards with "Got Your Banana Ice Cream Today?" instead of "Get Your Cheap Hot Dogs Here!" Imagine never feeling weird explaining what raw food is, no matter where you go. A juicer instead of a coffeemaker in every office, a little package of sprouts at every convenience store. . . . This sounds like a fantasy, yet we are the ones who can create it.

Another important way of supporting beginners in the raw-food movement is to prepare delicious meals for raw-food potlucks. Through these potlucks, you may introduce delicious raw food to many people, and you can literally influence people to make life-changing choices. Even if you eat simply now, don't just bring a couple of kale leaves to a potluck. I encourage you to take your time, spend an extra $10–$15, and prepare an attractive and yummy plate. I remember one of the first raw-food potlucks in my life, where the attendees brought plain salads and bowls of whole fruits. The most prepared dish was sliced bananas with toothpicks in them. There were several newcomers, curious about raw food, and I felt sorry for them when I saw their disappointed faces. Since then, I always try to bring two or three special dishes to every potluck I attend.

Please think about a raw-food teacher who impressed you most in your life. What was special about this teacher? Was he or she a dynamic speaker? Have you felt as if this teacher was your friend and you could trust her? Think for a moment with gratitude about this teacher, the one who touched your heart.

Now perhaps it's *your* turn to become a teacher. I've heard many raw-fooders say that they would like to become teachers. I believe that every single person in the world is a teacher, in potential, when they sincerely do what they love. Then they don't even have to advertise—those who want to will follow them and their path. While educating others, try carefully not to scare but to inspire your listeners, as fear is a destructive emotion. From my own observations, I know that staying on a diet out of fear is temporary and might last merely a couple of days.

I used to think that we teach mostly by example, and now I know that we teach *only* by example. I would like to inspire you to become and stay a living example. How many people do you think you will influence in your life by simply eating healthy? Think of all the people you touch in a day: all your neighbors, relatives, co-workers, and people who see you buying and eating healthy food. The cashier at your local store might ask, "Do you have a horse?" Perhaps you might reply, "No, but I have a juicer." The cashier wonders, "Maybe I should get one too." Even the other shoppers, when they see your green-purple-red-radiant-colored cart, might run quickly to the produce section and grab an additional head of romaine lettuce. When your children go to school and tell their teacher, "In our family we eat salad every day," don't they influence even the teacher? If your neighbor persistently invites you for a barbecue, and you keep showing up with a plate of "neat-balls" and a raw cake, they will inevitably begin to include more fresh foods in their menus.

Your co-workers may be eating fast food for lunch. They will notice your cute-looking raw snacks and most of all, your fresh look after every lunch break while they might feel tired and sleepy. People always subconsciously make the connection in their mind between a healthy glow and a healthy food choice. Your example will move them towards making a better choice for their health.

Your relatives could be the toughest challenge. They won't hesitate to let you know what they think. However, don't get discouraged too quickly. They could be the splinter in your side for the longest time, but at the same time they will be proud of you and even call you for advice, especially if they see your persistence. I remember how my father would always burst into angry accusations and criticism towards my dieting when I mentioned anything about raw food. Later, I would be shocked to learn from my aunt that my father had called her right after talking to me, confiding that he was eating 50% raw and sounding very proud of his daughter. Another relative of mine makes such a disgusted face every time I mention the benefits of raw food that I feel ridiculed. Then later, his wife tells me that he demanded raw salad for lunch. The initial negative reactions usually come from your loved ones as an attempt to defend themselves from the unknown. As you learned in Step 4, try to be a positive example instead of attempting to change others.

When you become a living example of the raw lifestyle, you literally influence thousands of people. Think of me, for example: what if I had not gone on the raw-food diet? What would have happened to all of my future students? Many of my former students are now making their living by teaching raw-food classes. You never know when the seed you have planted is going to germinate, sprout, and then blossom forth to inspire others. How many people can you influence in your lifetime directly and indirectly? Eventually, I think, the whole planet. *Is it worth a try?*

Part 4

RECIPES

Raw Family Green Smoothies

Below are five green smoothie recipes. They are merely basic ideas for your green creations. Feel free to substitute your own choice of greens and fruits for the ingredients. Enjoy!

Apple–Kale–Lemon

4 apples

1/2 lemon (juice only)

5 leaves of kale (remove white stems for better taste)

2 cups water

Peach–Spinach

6 peaches

2 handfuls of spinach leaves

2 cups water

Mango–Weeds

2 mangos

1 handful of edible weeds, such as lambsquarters, stinging nettles, purslane, etc.

2 cups water

Strawberry–Banana–Romaine

1 cup strawberries

2 bananas

1/2 bunch romaine, or 6–7 large leaves

2 cups water

Pear–Chard–Mint

4 ripe pears

5 leaves of chard

1/2 bunch mint

2 cups water

Each of these recipes makes 3 cups of green smoothie.

Raw Family Green Soup

1 large handful of greens (kale, spinach, chard, or any other)

1 bell pepper with seeds (or 2 tomatoes, or 1 cucumber)

Juice of two or three lemons

1/2 large (or one whole small) avocado

Add water as needed and blend to a desired consistency. We like to eat this soup with dulse leaves, grated carrot, or sprouts.

Serves 3–4.

Valya's Stupendously Magnificent, Outstandingly Exceptional, Green Spinach Soup

3 small avocados (or one extra large)

2 red bell peppers

1/2 bunch cilantro

1/2 bunch spinach

2 small lemons (peeled, without seeds)

2 cups pure water

1 small jalapeño pepper

1/2 teaspoon Celtic sea salt (optional)

Put all the ingredients in a Vita-Mix blender and blend well using the tamper. Once the ingredients are well blended, pour the soup into a large bowl. Add thinly sliced napa cabbage or red cabbage and dulse leaves or flakes.

Serves 6.

Real Rawssian Borscht

Blend these ingredients well in a blender:

2 cups water

3 beets

1 small ginger root (slice it first)

1–2 large cloves garlic

5–6 bay leaves

Pour the mixture into a big bowl.

Blend the following ingredients for a short time (about 30 seconds):

2 cups water

2 carrots

2 stalks celery

2 tablespoons apple cider vinegar

3–4 oranges, peeled, with seeds removed (seeds will make a very bitter taste)

1 tablespoon raw agave nectar

1/2 cup olive oil

Celtic sea salt to taste (optional)

Add 1/2 cup walnuts and blend on low speed very quickly, so the nuts break into small pieces but are not blended. Pour in the same bowl and stir.

DICE OR GRATE:

1/4 head cabbage

1–2 carrots

1 bunch parsley

Add grated ingredients to the blended mixture. Stir and serve.

Serves 7–10.

Generic Recipe for Chowder

Blend 1 cup cashews or walnuts with 1 cup water in blender until smooth.

Add the following and blend well:

1 cup water

1/4 cup olive oil

2–3 dates, pitted

1 cup chopped celery

Hot peppers to taste

1–2 cloves garlic

Celtic sea salt to taste (optional)

Now you have plain chowder. *Pick the flavor:*

For clam-chowder taste add: dulse flakes

For broccoli: chopped broccoli

For mushroom: your favorite mushrooms, dry or fresh

For tomato: chopped tomato

For carrot: grated carrots

For corn: cut corn off the cob or use frozen corn

For pea: fresh or frozen peas

Your own creation . . . Sprinkle with dry parsley flakes before serving.

Serves 5.

Chili

Blend the following ingredients in a blender:

1 cup water

2 cups fresh tomatoes, chopped

1/2 cup dates or raisins

1 cup sun-dried tomatoes

1 cup dehydrated mushrooms (optional)

1 cup chopped celery

2 tablespoons olive oil

Celtic sea salt to taste (optional)

1–2 tablespoons spaghetti seasoning

1–2 tablespoons juice of lime or lemon

Hot peppers to taste (optional)

2 cloves garlic

1 bunch basil

Add a half-pound of bean, pea, or lentil sprouts. Don't blend! Sprinkle with dry parsley flakes before serving.

Serves 5–7.

Gazpacho

Blend the following ingredients in a blender until smooth:

1/2 cup water

2 tablespoons olive oil

5 large ripe tomatoes

2 cloves garlic or spicy pepper to taste

5–7 dates, pitted (raisins work just as well)

1/4 cup lemon juice

1/2 teaspoon Celtic sea salt (optional)

1 bunch fresh basil

Now you have the gazpacho liquid.

Cut the following vegetables into 1/4-inch cubes:

1 large avocado

1 medium bell pepper

5 sticks celery

1 small onion (optional)

Mix all ingredients in a bowl and sprinkle with chopped parsley.

Serves 4–5.

I Can't Believe It's Just Cabbage

1 head white cabbage

2 tablespoons olive oil

1 teaspoon salt

1 lemon, squeezed (optional)

1 tablespoon nutritional yeast (optional)

Mix all ingredients in a bowl and decorate with your favorite herb.

Serves 5.

Igor's Crackers

Grind 2 cups flaxseed in a dry Vita-Mix container.

Blend together:

1 cup water

3 large carrots, chopped

3 stalks celery, chopped

4 cloves garlic (medium)

2 tomatoes (optional)

1 teaspoon caraway seed

1 teaspoon coriander seed

1 teaspoon Celtic sea salt (optional)

Mix ground flaxseed into blended mix by hand. Cover the dough with cheesecloth or a towel and let sit in a bowl at a warm room temperature overnight to ferment slightly.

Using a spatula, spread on non-stick dehydrating sheets. Divide into squares of desired size.

Dehydrate only until dry, but not crispy if you want it to taste like bread. Dry the mixture well for crispy crackers that will keep for a couple of months.

Makes 25–32 crackers.

Live Garden Burgers

Grind 1 pound of your favorite nuts or seeds in a food processor. Remove ground nuts to a bowl. Then combine the following ingredients and grind in a food processor:

1 pound carrots (or carrot pulp left after juicing carrots)

1 medium onion

1 tablespoon sweetener (agave nectar, dates, or raisins)

1 tablespoon oil

1–2 tablespoons poultry seasoning (or other herb seasoning)

Celtic sea salt to taste (optional)

If the mixture is not firm enough, add one or two of the following thickeners: dried dill weed, dried garlic, dried onion, dried parsley flakes, ground flaxseeds.

Form into balls, cutlets, or fillets and sprinkle with paprika shortly before serving.

Note: If you want "fish" burgers, add seaweed (dulse, kelp, or other seaweed) to the mixture.

Serves 10.

Live Burgers, Low-Fat Version

Grind 1 pound of sunflower seeds in a food processor.

Combine ground sunflower seeds with the following ingredients in a large bowl and mix well with your hands:

2 pounds carrot pulp (from juice or grated and squeezed)

2 pounds celery pulp (from juice or grated and squeezed)

1 medium onion, grated and squeezed

2 tablespoons sweetener (agave nectar, very ripe banana, or raisins, blended with a little water to the consistency of jam)

3 lemons, juiced

3 tablespoons olive oil

1–2 jalapeños or other spice to taste

1 teaspoon poultry seasoning

1/2 teaspoon Celtic sea salt (optional)

Mix well. You have to experiment to get the desired consistency. Shape into burgers—you may want to use an ice-scream scoop to make nice uniform shapes. Serve the burgers on lettuce leaves, crackers, or on the side with a salad.

This pâté will keep for at least one week in the fridge.

Makes 24 burgers.

Live Fries

Peel and slice one large jicama so it looks like French fries.

Combine in a bowl with:

1 tablespoon onion powder

2 tablespoons olive oil

1 tablespoon paprika

Sea salt to taste

We recommend serving Live Fries with Tomato Basil Sauce (please see below).

Serves 5.

Tomato Basil Sauce

Blend 2 cups fresh chopped tomatoes.

Add the following ingredients to the blended fresh tomatoes and blend:

1 cup sun-dried tomatoes

3/4 cup chopped fresh basil

Juice of 1 medium lemon

2 tablespoons olive oil

4 dates (or some raisins)

1–2 cloves garlic

Serves 9.

Live Pizza

CRUST:

Grind 2 cups flaxseed in a dry Vita-Mix container or in a coffee grinder.

Blend together:

3 stalks celery, chopped

2 medium tomatoes

1 cup water

1 large onion, chopped

1 teaspoon Celtic sea salt (optional)

Mix ground flaxseed into blended mix by hand. Spread on dehydrating sheets with a spatula. Divide into squares of desired size. Dehydrate only until dry but not crispy.

TOPPING:

Blend the following ingredients with as little water as possible:

2 cups sunflower seeds

1/2 cup sun-dried tomatoes

1/2 cup raisins

Juice of 1 medium lemon

2 tablespoons olive oil

1 tablespoon dry basil

Pour in a bowl. Add:

1 tablespoon dry onion

1 tablespoon dry garlic

2 tablespoons nutritional yeast

1 tablespoon miso

Mix well.

MAKING PIZZA:

Spread topping on squares of crust. Decorate with grated yams, sliced cherry tomatoes, sliced mushrooms, sliced olives, and chopped parsley.

Makes 12 "slices" of pizza.

Nori Rolls

For this recipe you will need:

5 raw nori sheets

PÂTÉ MIXTURE:

1/2 cup walnuts

2 cups sunflower seeds, soaked overnight

3 garlic cloves

1 cup chopped celery

1 teaspoon Celtic sea salt (optional)

2 tablespoons olive oil

1/2 cup lemon juice

1 teaspoon curry powder (or your favorite seasoning)

Slice the following ingredients into long thin strips:

Half an avocado

Half a large bell pepper

2 green onions

Blend all the pâté ingredients in a food processor until creamy. Spread the pâté onto a sheet of nori and add the thinly sliced vegetables. Roll up tight in nori sheet. (Note: To make the nori sheets stick better you can moisten them a little with water, lemon, tomato, or orange juice.) Let the nori rolls sit for 10 minutes and then begin slicing them into 2-inch slices.

Makes 15–20 nori rolls.

Nut or Seed Cheese

2 cups any nuts or seeds, soaked overnight

1 1/2 cups water

Soak the nuts and seeds in water overnight. Drain and rinse. Put into blender with one cup of water and blend well to break the nuts down into a fine cream. Pour into sprout bag. Hang the sprout bag over a sink or bowl (to drain off the whey) and let ferment at room temperature for approximately 8–12 hours.

Transfer cheese to a bowl, mix with your favorite seasonings, and stir well. To flavor seed cheese you may use any combination of the following: garlic, lemon juice, chopped fresh cilantro, curry powder, chopped or dry parsley, chopped or dry dill, sun-dried tomatoes, chopped scallions, basil, olive oil, and Celtic sea salt.

Makes 1 pint. Keeps for at least 7 days in a covered container in the refrigerator.

Valya's Spicy Almond Cheese

Mix the following ingredients in a bowl:

2 cups pulp from almond milk (pulp should not be sweetened)

2 tablespoons olive oil

1/2 cup lemon juice

1/2 teaspoon Celtic sea salt (optional)

1/4 cup fresh or dried dill weed

1/2 cup diced onions

1/2 cup diced red bell pepper

Decorate with cherry tomatoes.

Serves 6.

Sunny Spread

2 cups sunflower seeds, soaked overnight

1/2 cup walnuts

1 cup chopped celery

2 tablespoons olive oil

1/2 cup lemon juice

1 tablespoon dry basil

2 cloves garlic

1 1/2 teaspoons Celtic sea salt (optional)

Blend ingredients in food processor until smooth.

Be creative and serve on a cracker, roll up in a cabbage leaf, or stuff a bell pepper.

Serves 12.

Sergei's Hummus

Blend the following ingredients in a food processor:

2 cups garbanzo beans, sprouted for 1 day

1 cup tomatoes, chopped

1 cup celery, chopped

2 tablespoons olive oil

1–2 tablespoons (dry) or 1 cup (fresh) dill or basil

1–2 tablespoons lime or lemon juice

Hot peppers to taste

Celtic sea salt to taste (optional)

2–3 cloves garlic

Sprinkle with dry parsley flakes before serving.

Serves 5–7.

Generic Cake Recipe

CRUST:

Combine the following ingredients, mixing well:

1 cup ground nuts or seeds

1 tablespoon oil

1 tablespoon raw agave nectar

OPTIONAL:

1/2 cup chopped or crushed fresh fruits or berries,
    or 1/2 cup dry fruits, soaked for 1–2 hours, then ground

1 teaspoon vanilla

1/2 teaspoon nutmeg

1/2 cup raw carob powder

Peel from 4 tangerines, well ground

If mixture is not firm enough, add psyllium husk or shredded coconut. Form into crust on a flat plate.

TOPPING:

Blend the following ingredients well; add water with a teaspoon if needed:

1/2 cup fresh or frozen fruit

1/2 cup nuts (white nuts look pretty)

2 tablespoons olive oil

2–3 tablespoons raw agave nectar

Juice of 1 medium lemon

1 teaspoon vanilla

Spread evenly over the crust. Decorate with fruits, berries, and nuts. Give your cake a name. Chill.

Serves 12.

Sergei's Young Coconut Dream Cake

This cake won a contest at the Portland Raw Food Festival.

CRUST:

1 cup raw unsoaked walnuts

1/2 cup of your favorite pitted dates

1/4 cup young coconut water

4 tablespoons raw carob

1 small papaya

Blend the walnuts and dates in a food processor until the mixture is smooth. Mix in the carob and the coconut water. Spread one layer of crust out on a plate. Place sliced papaya on top of first layer. Place second layer of nuts and dates on top.

ICING:

1 cup young coconut meat

Water, enough to blend into thick topping

1 tablespoon raw agave nectar

Blend all the ingredients in a Vita-Mix. Spread icing on cake. Decorate with fruit slices and nuts.

Serves 12.

Un-Chocolate Cake

CRUST:

Combine the following ingredients, mixing well:

1 cup nuts, ground

1 cup raisins

1 cup raw carob powder

1 cup prunes, soaked 1–2 hours and ground

1 tablespoon oil

1 teaspoon Frontier brand butterscotch flavor

1 teaspoon vanilla

1/2 teaspoon nutmeg or Nama Shoyu soy sauce

Peel from 4 tangerines, well ground

Form into one-inch layer on a flat plate. Spread ground prunes between layers (form as many layers as you want).

TOPPING:

Blend the following ingredients well; add water with a teaspoon if needed:

1 cup ripe avocado meat

1 teaspoon olive oil

3 tablespoons raw agave nectar

Juice of 1 medium lemon

1 teaspoon vanilla

4–5 tablespoons raw carob powder

Spread evenly over the crust, or squeeze using a decorating bag. Garnish with fruits, berries, and nuts. Chill.

Serves 12.

Sergei's Amazing Truffles

1 cup walnuts

1/2 cup of your favorite pitted dates

1/4 cup young coconut water

4 tablespoons raw carob

Blend the walnuts and dates in a food processor until the mixture is smooth.

Mix the carob and coconut water. Shape the mixture into small balls and roll in carob. Decorate with your favorite fruit.

Makes 8–12 truffles.

Alla's Cranberry Scones

2 cups grated apples

2 cups carrot pulp, left over from making carrot juice

2 cups raisins or chopped dates

1 cup cranberries (fresh or dry)

2 cups almonds, ground

1 cup flaxseed blended with 1 cup water

2 tablespoons raw agave nectar

3 tablespoons olive oil

Mix with hands. You have to experiment to get the consistency desired. Drop by spoonfuls onto teflex sheets. Dehydrate at 105–115° for several hours: approximately 4 hours on one side, then flip and dehydrate for 3 hours on the opposite side.

Makes 24 scones.

Sergei's Butternut Squash Cookies

4 cups peeled butternut squash, chopped into medium-sized chunks

1 cup raisins

Juice of one orange

1/2 teaspoon nutmeg

1 teaspoon cinnamon

3 tablespoons raw agave nectar

Blend the chopped squash in a food processor and transfer into a bowl. Next blend the raisins and the orange juice in a food processor and add to the squash mixture. Add the rest of the ingredients to the bowl and mix thoroughly.

Use an ice-cream scoop and scoop the mixture onto a dehydrator tray. Flatten each cookie to a thickness of one inch. Set the dehydrator for 105° and leave in 12–15 hours.

Makes 7–11 cookies.

Sesame Cookies

A fabulous way to use all leftover sesame pulp after making sesame milk.

5 cups sesame seed pulp

2 cups raisins

Juice of one orange

3 tablespoons raw agave nectar

Poppy seeds to garnish

Blend raisins and orange juice in food processor until mixture is finely pureed. Add to a bowl with the sesame seed pulp. Add agave nectar and mix thoroughly.

Spread the mixture onto non-sticking dehydrator sheets and cut into squares, using a spatula. Sprinkle with poppy seeds and set in the dehydrator at 105°. Dehydrate 12–15 hours or until dry.

Makes 15–20 cookies.

Morning Cereal

Soak 1 cup oat groats overnight.

Blend with 3/4 cup water.

Add 1/4 cup dates without pits (or use raisins) and blend.

Add 1 teaspoon of your favorite oil (optional).

Add Celtic sea salt to taste (optional).

Garnish with fresh fruits and berries before serving.

Serves 3.

Nut or Seed Milk

1 cup any nuts or seeds, soaked overnight

2 cups pure water

2–3 dates

1/4 teaspoon Celtic sea salt (optional)

Blend all ingredients thoroughly in a blender until smooth.
Strain mixture through a nut milk bag or sprout bag.
Pour into a jar.

Serves 4.

Notes

Part One: Why Raw Food?

Chapter 1

1. J. Whittaker, *Reversing Diabetes* (New York: Warner Books, 1990).

Chapter 3

1. Weston A. Price, *Nutrition and Physical Degeneration*, 6th Edition (La Mesa, CA: The Price-Pottenger Nutrition Foundation, Inc., 2003).

2. Ibid.

Chapter 4

1. For further information contact: Lars Christensen, Department of Food Science, Research Centre Aarslev, Denmark. Tel.: +45 8999 3367; e-mail: LarsP.Christensen@agrsci.dk.

2. A. Waladkhani and M. Clemens, "Effect of dietary phytochemicals on cancer development," *International Journal of Molecular Medicine*, Germany, 1998.

3. R. Sinha et al., "Development of a food frequency questionnaire module and databases for compounds in cooked and processed meats," *Acta Phisiol Scand* 130(3):467–74 (July 1987). Nutrition Epidemiology Branch, Division of Cancer, Epidemiology and Genetics, National Cancer Institute, Bethesda, MD 20892-7273, USA. sinhar@nih.gov.

4. Summary—Acrylamide in Heat-Processed Foods. Livsmedelsverket, Swedish National Food Administration, Stockholm, April 2002.

5. L. Link and J. Potter, "Diseases associated with raw versus cooked vegetables and cancer risk," *Cancer Epidemiology Biomarkers Preview* 13(9):1422–35 (September 2004).

6. J. Alexander, "Chemical and biological properties related to toxicity of heated fats," *Environ Health* 7(1):125–38 (January 1981).

7. K. Wu. "Meat mutagens and risk of distal colon adenoma in a cohort of U.S. men," *Cancer Epidemiology Biomarkers Preview* 15(6):1120–25 (June 2006).

8. K. Steinmetz and J. Potter, *Vegetables, fruit, and cancer prevention: a review.* World Cancer Research Fund, London, England.

9. I. Romieu and C. Trenga, *Diet and obstructive lung disease.* Pan American Health Organization and National Institute of Public Health, Center for Population Studies, Cuernavaca, Morelos, Mexico.

10. M. Morris et al., "Associations of vegetable and fruit consumption with age-related cognitive change," *Neurology* 67:1370–76 (2006).

11. T. Goldberg, MS RD, et al., "Advanced Glycoxidation End Products in Commonly Consumed Foods," *American Dietetic Assoc. Journal* 105(4):647 (April 2005).

12. Ravichandran Ramasamy et al., "Advanced glycation end products and RAGE: a common thread in aging, diabetes, neurodegeneration, and inflammation." Department of Pathology, Columbia University Medical Center, New York, March 7, 2005.

13. C. Borek, PhD, "AGE Breakers," *LE Magazine*, August 2001.

14. F. Tessier, "Structure and Mechanism of Formation of Human Lens Fluorophore LM-1," *J Biol Chem* 274(30):20796–20804 (July 23, 1999).

15. Glutathione (GSH) http://www.vitimmune.com/1-skin_antioxidants_letter.htm.

16. T. Goldberg et al. See note 11 above.

17. J. Uribarri, M. Peppa, W. Cai, T. Goldberg, M. Lu, H. Vlassara, "Restriction of glycotoxins markedly reduces AGE toxins in renal failure patients," *J Am Soc Nephrol* 14:728–31 (2003).

18. G. Cousens, MD, MD (H). EWellness Articles with Dr. Cousens. http://www.treeoflife.nu/articles.html.

19. http://awi.vlaanderen.be/documenten/COST_927_MoU_TA_3rd.pdf.

Chapter 5

1. Wikipedia, the free encyclopedia on the Internet, http://en.wikipedia.org/wiki/Life.

2. Dr. Tom Lonsdale, "Optimum Animal Nutrition and Complementary and Alternative Therapies in Veterinary Medicine," *British Journal of Small Animal Practice* (December 1995). http://www.shirleys-wellness-cafe.com.

3. http://www.shirleys-wellness-cafe.com.

Chapter 6

1. *The Dangers of Aspirin & NSAIDS*. American College of Gastroenterology. Bethesda, MD, 2006.

2. Coordinating Center for Infectious Diseases, Division of Bacterial and Mycotic Diseases. Atlanta, GA, publication dated October 24, 2005.

Chapter 7

1. Human Prehistory. Anistoriton, an electronic *Journal of History,* 2005. http://users.hol.gr/~dilos/prehis.htm.

2. N. Boauz, *Quarry: Closing in on the Missing Link* (New York: The Free Press, 1993).

3. "Rainforest," Microsoft® Encarta® Online Encyclopedia 2006, http://encarta.msn.com © 1997–2006 Microsoft Corporation.

4. D. Johanson and B. Edgar, *From Lucy to Language* (New York: Simon & Schuster, 1996).

5. D. Moerman, *Native American Ethnobotany* (Portland, OR: Timber Press, 1998).

6. Tallyrand, *History of Cooking.* New Zealand: Tallyrand's Culinary Fare, 2005.

7. http://www.clover.okstate.edu/fourh/aitc/lessons/extras/facts/wheat.html#history.

8. T. D. Price, *Europe's First Farmers* (Madison, WI: University of Wisconsin, 2000).

9. Kansas Foundation for Agriculture in Classroom, KSU, 2004.

10. Tallyrand, *History of Cooking.* See note 6 above.

11. http://history.enotes.com/guides/history-topics.

12. Tolstoi, L. *War and Peace* (New York: Classic Books, 2003).

13. Goethe, J. *Italian Journey: 1786–1788* (New York: Penguin Classics, 1992).

14. C. Hieatt, *Curye on Inglysch: Middle English Recipes: English Culinary Manuscripts of the Fourteenth Century.* Oxford, UK: Early English Text Society, 1985.

15. Translation by James L. Matterer, *Gode Cookery* (Clinton, PA: Gode Cookery Recipe Collection, 2005). www.godecookery.com.

Chapter 8

1. P. Rincon, "Early human fire skills revealed." BBC News, 2006. http://news.bbc.co.uk/go/pr/fr/-/2/hi/science/nature/3670017.stm.

2. http;//www.hbci.com/~wenonah/new/howfindv.htm.

3. Tallyrand, *History of Cooking*. New Zealand: Tallyrand's Culinary Fare, 2005.

4. Wikipedia, the free encyclopedia on the Internet, http://en.wikipedia.org/wiki/Sugar.

5. Wikipedia, the free encyclopedia on the Internet, http://en.wikipedia.org/wiki/Canning.

6. *U.S. News and World Report*, December 27, 1999.

7. http://seer.cancer.gov.

8. Benjamin Harrow, *Casimir Funk: Pioneer in Vitamins and Hormones* (New York: Dodd, Mead & Company, 1955).

9. K. Carpenter. *A Short History of Nutritional Science* (Bristol, UK: The British Journal of Nutrition, 2003).

10. H. Magee, "Application of Nutrition to Public Health: Some Lessons of the War. 1946," *British Med. Journal*, issue #475-481.

Chapter 10

1. Wikipedia, the free encyclopedia on the Internet, http://en.wikipedia.org/wiki/Soil_life.

2. Vyapaka Dasa, organic farm inspector, *It Ain't Just Dirt!* Canada, 2005. Posted at: http://www.hkrl.com/soils.html.

3. P. Tompkins and C. Bird, *Secrets of the Soil* (Anchorage, AK: Earthpulse Press Inc., 2002).

4. D. Blume, "Food and Permaculture." Article at: http://www.permaculture.com/permaculture/About_Permaculture/food.shtml.

5. Ibid.

6. L. Kervran, *Biological Transmutations* (London: Crosby Lockwood, 1972).

Part Two: Human Dependency on Cooked Food

Chapter 11

1. W. Price, D.D.S., *Nutrition and Physical Degeneration* (La Mesa, CA: The Price-Pottenger Nutrition Foundation, Inc., 2003).

2. T. Turpin, Entomologist. *Bug du jour.* "Down the Garden Path." Cooperative Extension Service, Purdue University, IN, 2004.

3. J. Allotey, "Utilization of Useful Insects as Food Source." Department of Biological Sciences, University of Botswana, Private Bag 0022, Gaborone, Botswana. Posted at: http://www.ajfand.net/Issue-V-files/IssueV-Short%20Communication%20-%20Allotey.htm.

4. M. Gelfand, *Diet and Tradition in an African Culture* (Edinburgh. UK: E and S Livingstone, 1971).

5. Posted at: http://news.nationalgeographic.com/news/2004/07/0715_040715_tvinsectfood.html.

6. S. Guynup and N. Ruggia. *For Most People, Eating Bugs Is Only Natural.* National Geographic Channel, July 15, 2004. Posted at: http://news.nationalgeographic.com/news/2004/07/0715_040715_tvinsectfood.html.

7. R. Kumar, *Insect Pests of Agriculture in Papua New Guinea. Part 1: Principles and Practice. Pests of tree crops and stored products.* UPNG Printery, Waigani. 2001: 723. Posted at: http://www.ajfand.net/Issue-V-files/IssueV-Short%20Communication%20-%20Allotey.htm.

8. W. Lyon, *Insects as Human Food (Microlivestock),* Ohio State University Extension Fact Sheet, Entomology, HYG-2160-96. Columbus, OH, 1996.

9. Ibid.

10. Dr. Joseph Mercola, "Vitamin B-12: Are You Getting It?" Posted at: http://www.mercola.com/2002/jan/30/vitamin_B-12_a.htm.

11. U.S. Department of Agriculture, Agricultural Research Service. 2003. USDA Nutrient Database for Standard Reference, Release 16. Nutrient Data Laboratory Home Page, http://www.nal.usda.gov/fnic/cgi-bin/nut_search.pl.

12. "The Food Defect Action Levels: Current Levels for Natural or Unavoidable Defects for Human Use that Present No Health Hazard." U.S. Department of Health & Human Services, 1989.

13. S. Guynup and N. Ruggia, *For Most People, Eating Bugs Is Only Natural.* See note 6 above.

14. Ibid.

15. Ibid.

Chapter 12

1. Weill Medical College of Cornell University, New York, 2006, an ongoing research report found on their website: "Addiction, Substance Dependence."

Chapter 13

1. J. Hirschmann and C. Munter, *Overcoming Overeating* (Robbinsdale, MN: Fawcett, 1998).

2. L. Eliot, *What's Going On In There? How the Brain and Mind Develop in the First Five Years of Life* (New York: Bantam Books, 1999).

3. E. Hess, *Imprinting* (New York: D. Van Nostrand Company, 1973).

4. Ibid.

5. Wellness International Network Ltd—http://web.winltd.com.

6. R. Holien, "Weight loss brings hope," *Argus Leader,* December 8, 2002. Sioux Falls, North Dakota.

7. http://www.rawreform.com.

Chapter 14

1. L. Eliot, *What's Going On In There? How the Brain and Mind Develop in the First Five Years of Life* (New York: Bantam Books, 1999).

2. H.C. Gore, "Formation of Maltose in Sweet Potatoes on Cooking," *Industrial and Engineering Chemistry,* Vol. 15, No. 9 (1923), Washington, DC.

3. J. Higdon, *Glycemic Index and Glycemic Load,* Oregon State University, 2005.

4. United States Department of Agriculture. http://www.usda.gov/factbook/chapter2.htm.

5. A. Kaplan, *Medical Issues and the Eating Disorders* (New York: Brunner/Mazel, 1993).

6. "Toasting the Toaster: The Original Comfort Food Remains a Breakfast Staple for Americans." Study conducted by Grain Foods Foundation in 2005. Rochester, NY. http://www.grainpower.org.

7. S. Fukudome, "Gluten exorphin C: A novel opioid peptide derived from wheat gluten," *FEBS Letters* 316(1):17–19 (1993).

8. F. Huebner, "Demonstration of high opioid-like activity in isolated peptides from wheat gluten hydrolysates," *Peptides* 5(6):1139–47 (1984).

9. E. Usdin et al., *Endorphins in Mental Health Research* (New York: Oxford University Press, 1979).

10. F. Huebner. See note 8 above.

11. G. Fanciulli et al., "Prolactin and growth hormone response to intracerebroventricular administration of the food opioid peptide gluten exorphin B5 in rats," *Life Sciences* 4(71):20 (2002), http://www.pubmed.gov.

12. U.S. Department of Agriculture, Agricultural Research Service. 2006. USDA National Nutrient Database for Standard Reference, Release 19. Nutrient Data Laboratory Home Page, http://www.ars.usda.gov/ba/bhnrc/ndl.

13. L. Cordain, *Cereal Grains: Humanity's Double-Edged Sword* (Fort Collins, CO: Department of Exercise and Sport Science, Colorado State University, 1999).

14. M. Froetschel, *Bioactive Peptides in Digesta That Regulate Gastrointestinal Function and Intake* (Athens, GA: Department of Animal and Dairy Science, University of Georgia, Athens, 2006).

15. T. Matsumoto, "Determination of mutagens, amino-alpha-carbolines in grilled foods and cigarette smoke condensate," *Cancer Letters* 12(1–2):105–10 (March 1981).

16. M. Kampa et al., "Identification of a novel opioid peptide (Tyr-Val-Pro-Phe-Pro) derived from human a_{S1} casein (a_{S1}-casomorphin), and a_{S1}-casomorphin amide," *Biochemical Journal* 319:903–08 (1996). Printed in Great Britain.

17. R. Kennedy, MD, *Addiction to Salt.* Posted at: http://www.medical-library.net.

Chapter 15

1. http://wordnet.princeton.edu.

2. http://www.bbc.co.uk/food/tv_and_radio/favouritefood_index.shtml.

Chapter 16

1. National Institute of Mental Health (NIMH), 2006, nimhinfo@nih.gov.

2. Australian Institute of Health and Welfare, *National Health Priority Areas Mental Health: A Report Focusing on Depression*, 1998.

3. Harvard University study reported in *Harvard Mental Health Newsletter*, February 2002.

4. World Health Organization (WHO) report quoted in BBC-Online, January 9, 2001.

5. Agency for Healthcare Research and Quality, *National Healthcare Quality Report*, 2003.

6. K. Kochanek et al., "Deaths: final data for 2002," *National Vital Statistics Reports* 12; 53 (5):1–115 (October 2004).

7. T. Walsh et al., "Placebo Response in Studies of Major Depression: Variable, Substantial, and Growing," *JAMA* 287:1840–47 (April 2002).

8. I. Kirsch, PhD, and D. Antonuccio, PhD, "Antidepressants Versus Placebos: Meaningful Advantages Are Lacking," *Psychiatric Times* 19:9 (2004).

9. B. Murray, "Getting to the Essential 'We' in Wellness," *Monitor on Psychology* 33(10) (November 2002).

10. H. Koenig et al., "Modeling the Cross-Sectional Relationships Between Religion, Physical Health, Social Support, and Depressive Symptoms," *American Journal of Geriatric Psychiatry* 5:131–43 (1997).

11. *Twelve Steps and Twelve Traditions* (New York: Alcoholics Anonymous World Services, 1990).

12. www.recoveringnurses.org.

13. *Merriam-Webster's Dictionary*, http://www.m-w.com.

14. C. Ringwald, *The Soul of Recovery: Uncovering the Spiritual Dimension in the Treatment of Addictions* (New York: Oxford University Press, USA, 2002).

15. A. Kohn, *The Brighter Side of Human Nature: Altruism and Empathy in Everyday Life* (New York: Basic Books, 1992).

Part Three: How to End Your Dependency on Cooked Food (The 12 Steps)

Step 1

1. Weill Medical College of Cornell University, New York, 2006, an ongoing research report found on their website: "Addiction, Substance Dependence."

Step 2

1. What's New in Health: February 2006 Archives. Posted at: http://www.foxnews.com/story/0,2933,185717,00.html.

Step 3

1. CBS News, "Report: Restaurants Should Go On Diet," Washington, June 2, 2006. http://www.cbsnews.com.

2. USDA, "Fruit and Tree Nuts Situation and Outlook Yearbook," 2000, and "Vegetables and Specialties Situation and Outlook Yearbook," 2000. www.ers.usda.gov.

3. E. Sloan, "News release, Institute of Food Technologists," *Food Technology,* January 6, 2006.

4. National Restaurant Association. "Restaurant Industry Fact Sheet 2006." http://www.restaurant.org.

5. S. Nelson, ABC News Homepage, "Good Morning America," August 8, 2005. http://abcnews.go.com.

6. K. Kane, Market Leadership. Franchise International, October 2006. http://www.franchise-international.net.

7. National Restaurant Association. See note 4 above.

8. http://www.wendys-invest.com/ne/wen092104.php.

Step 4

1. M. Rosenberg, *Nonviolent Communication: A Language of Life* (Encinitas, CA: Puddledancer Press, 2003).

Step 5

1. *Merriam-Webster Online Dictionary,* http://www.m-w.com.

2. Y. Zhang and A. Fishbach, "The Dilution Model: How Additional Goals Undermine the Perceived Instrumentality of a Shared Path," *Journal of Personality and Social Psychology,* University of Chicago, 2006.

3. A. Fishbach and J. Shah, "Self Control in Action: Implicit Dispositions toward Goals and Away from Temptations," *Journal of Personality and Social Psychology,* University of Chicago, 2006.

Step 6

1. Homer, *The Odyssey* (New York: Farrar, Straus and Giroux, 1998).

Step 7

1. A. Emmons and M. McCullough, *The Psychology of Gratitude* (New York: Oxford University Press, 2004).

2. E. Polak and M. McCullough, "Is Gratitude an Alternative to Materialism?" *Journal of Happiness Studies,* 2006, DOI 10.1007/s10902-005-3649-5.

3. T. Kasser, *The High Price of Materialism* (Cambridge, MA: The MIT Press, 2002).

4. M. McCullough, S. Kilpatrick, R. Emmons, and D. Larson, "Is gratitude a moral affect?" *Psychological Bulletin* 127 (2001).

5. J. Hughes and C. Stoney, "Depressed mood is related to high-frequency heart rate variability during stressors," *Psychosomatic Medicine* 62:796–803 (2000).

6. M. McCullough, S. Sandage, and E. Worthington, *To Forgive Is Human: How to Put Your Past in the Past* (Westmont, IL: InterVarsity Press, 1997).

7. M. McCullough, P. Orsulak, A. Brandon, and L. Akers, "Rumination, Fear and Cortisol: An In Vivo Study of Interpersonal Transgressions," *Health Psychology,* 2006.

Step 9

1. R. Lyons, "Scientists Find Even Mild Exercise Prolongs Life," *The New York Times,* July 27, 1984.

2. J. McDougall, "Sunny Days, Keeping Those Clouds Away." Posted at: www.drmcdougall.com.

3. A. Vasquez, G. Manso, J. Cannell, "The Clinical Importance of Vitamin D: A Paradigm Shift with Implications for All Healthcare Providers," *Alternative Therapies in Health and Medicine* 10(5):28–36; quiz 37, 94 (Sep-Oct 2004).

4. R. Stein, "Vitamin D Deficiency Called Major Health Risk," *Washington Post,* May 21, 2004.

5. E. Kellogg, "Air ions: Their possible biological significance and effects," *J Bioelectricity* 3 (1984).

6. M. White, *The Way You Breathe Can Make You Sick or Make You Well.* E-book. Available at: www.breathing.com.

7. F. Batmanghelidj, *Your Body's Many Cries for Water* (Falls Church, VA: Global Health Solutions, 1997).

8. R. Sapolsky, *Why Zebras Don't Get Ulcers* (New York: Owl Books, 2004).

9. *How to Reduce Stress: Suggestions to College Students.* State University of New York at Buffalo. Posted at: http://ub-counseling.buffalo.edu/stress-management.shtml.

10. http://www.victorianturkishbath.org/2HISTORY/3CLOSER.htm.

11. Grenader A.B.—"Impact of Cold Tempering and Winter Swimming on Human Organism," Second scientific and methodological conference on cold tempering and winter swimming, Minsk, 1967 (in Russian).

12. Kondakova-Varlamova, *Methods of Tempering Procedures,* 1980 (in Russian).

13. G. Malakhov, *Tempering and Healing with Water* (Moscow: Stalker Publishing, 2006; in Russian).

14. E. Maistrakh, *Physiological Pathology of Cooling of Human Organism* (Moscow: Medicine Publishing, 1975; in Russian).

15. A. Kolgushkin, *Tempering* (Moscow: Ripol Classic Publishing, 1997; in Russian).

16. A. Chizhevsky, *The Terrestrial Echo of Solar Storms* (Moscow: Mysl Publishing, 1976). Translated into English.

17. A. Baranov and V. Kidalov, *Healing with Cold* (Kemerovo, Russia: Astrel Publishing, 2000; in Russian).

18. M. Alexsandrov, *Human Safety on the Sea* (St. Petersburg, Russia: Sudostroenie Publishing, 1983; in Russian).

19. V. Grebyonkin, "Report of the President of The Federation of Tempering and Winter Swimming." Posted at: http://umcsa.narod.ru/rus/index.htm and http://www.russianrecords.ru/index.php?option=com_content&task =view&id=18.

20. Vancouver Polar Bear Swim Club, http://www.city.vancouver.bc.ca/ parks/events/polarbear.

21. R. Zhbankov, *The Tasks and Perspectives of Cold Tempering and Winter Swimming*. Second Scientific and Methodological Conference on Cold Tempering and Winter Swimming, Minsk, 1967 (in Russian).

22. Ibid.

Step 11

1. D. Trebichavska, *Depression*. Phoenix, 2005. Posted at: http://www.health-transformations.net/depression.htm.

Bibliography

Batmanghelidj, F. *Your Body's Many Cries for Water.* Falls Church, VA: Global Health Solutions, 1997.

Boauz, N. *Quarry: Closing in on the Missing Link.* New York: The Free Press, 1993.

Boutenko, V. *Green for Life.* Ashland, OR: Raw Family Publishing, 2005.

Boutenko, V., Boutenko, I., Boutenko, S., and Boutenko, V. *Raw Family: A True Story of Awakening.* Ashland, OR: Raw Family Publishing, 2005.

Eliot, L. *What's Going On In There? How the Brain and Mind Develop in the First Five Years of Life.* New York: Bantam Books, 1999.

Emmons, A., and McCullough, M. *The Psychology of Gratitude.* New York: Oxford University Press, 2004.

Fuller, R. *Critical Path.* New York: St. Martin's Press, 1981.

Goethe, J. *Italian Journey: 1786–1788.* New York: Penguin Classics, 1992.

Hess, E. *Imprinting.* New York: D. Van Nostrand Company, 1973.

Homer, *The Odyssey.* New York: Farrar, Straus and Giroux, 1998.

Johanson, D., and Edgar, B. *From Lucy to Language.* New York: Simon & Schuster, 1996.

Kaplan, A. *Medical Issues and the Eating Disorders.* New York: Brunner & Mazel, 1993.

Kervran, L. *Biological Transmutations.* London: Crosby Lockwood, 1972.

Kohn, A. *The Brighter Side of Human Nature: Altruism and Empathy in Everyday Life.* New York: Basic Books, 1992.

McCullough, M. *Forgiveness: Theory, Research, and Practice.* New York: Guilford Press, 2000.

McCullough, M. *To Forgive is Human: How to Put Your Past in the Past.* Downers Grove, IL: InterVarsity Press, 1997.

Moerman, D. *Native American Ethnobotany.* Portland, OR: Timber Press, 1998.

Munter, C. *Overcoming Overeating.* Robbinsdale, MN: Fawcett, 1998.

Murray, B. *Creating Optimism.* New York: McGraw-Hill, 2004.

Post, S., et al. *Altruism & Love*. Philadelphia: Templeton Foundation Press, 2003.

Price, W., DDS. *Nutrition and Physical Degeneration*. La Mesa, CA: The Price-Pottenger Nutrition Foundation, Inc., 2003.

Ringwald, C. *The Soul of Recovery: Uncovering the Spiritual Dimension in the Treatment of Addictions*. Oxford: Oxford University Press, 2002.

Rosenberg, M. *Nonviolent Communication: A Language of Life*. Encinitas, CA: Puddledancer Press, 2003.

Sapolsky, R. *Why Zebras Don't Get Ulcers*. New York: Owl Books, 2004.

Stokes, A. *Raw Reform: Revealing the Physical Changes*. www.rawreform.com, 2006.

Tolstoi, L. *War and Peace*. New York: Classic Books, 2003.

Tompkins, P., and Bird, C. *Secrets of the Soil*. Anchorage, AK: Earthpulse Press Inc., 2002.

Twelve Steps and Twelve Traditions. Alcoholics Anonymous World Services. New York, 1990.

Whittaker, J. *Reversing Diabetes*. New York: Warner Books, 1990.

Index